VITALITY SUPREME

BY
BERNARR
MACFADDEN

DISCLAIMER

The exercises and advice contained within this book is for educational and entertainment purposes only. The exercises described may be too strenuous or dangerous for some people, and the reader should consult with a physician before engaging in any of them.

The author and publisher of this book are not responsible in any manner whatsoever for any injury, which may occur through the use or misuse of the information presented here.

Vitality Supreme originally published in 1915

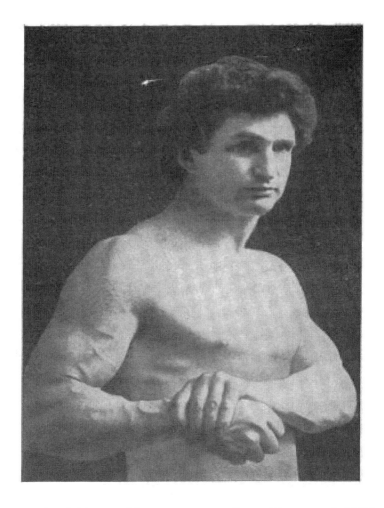

Bernarr Macfadden at thirty-two years of age. Photograph 1900.

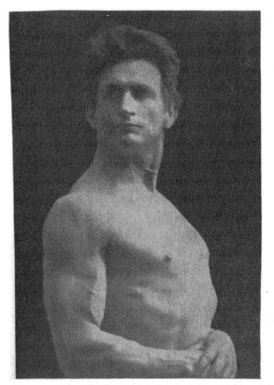

A recent photograph of Bernarr Macfadden, after thirty years of physical culture. Compared with the previous photograph it shows that at forty-seven the author of this book is in as perfect physical condition as in his early thirties.

PREFACE

The war cry of to-day in peace no less than in war is for efficiency. We need stronger, more capable men; healthier, superior women. Force is supreme-the king of all mankind. And it is force that stands back of efficiency, for efficiency, first of all, means power. It comes from power, and power either comes directly from inheritance or it is developed by an intelligent application of the laws that control the culture of the physique. The value of efficiency is everywhere recognized. The great prizes of life come only to those who are efficient. Those who desire capacities of this sort must recognize the importance of a strong, enduring physique. The body must be developed completely, splendidly. The buoyancy, vivacity, energy, enthusiasm and ambition ordinarily associated with youth can be maintained through middle age and in some cases even to old age. If your efforts are to be crowned with the halo of success, they must be spurred on by the pulsating throbbing powers that accompany physical excellence. These truly extraordinary characteristics come without effort to but few of us, but they can be developed, attained and maintained.

Why not throb with superior vitality! Why not possess the physical energy of a young lion? For then you will compel success. You will stand like a wall if need be, or rush with the force of a charging bison towards the desired achievements. This book sends forth a message of paramount importance to those who need added efficiency. Adherence to the principles laid down herein will add to the characteristics that insure splendid achievements. They will increase the power of your body and mind and soul. They will help each human entity to become a live personality. They will enable you to live fully, joyously. They will help you to feel, enjoy, suffer, every moment of each day. It is only when you are thus thrilled with the eternal force of life that you reach the highest pinnacle of attainable capacities and powers. Hidden forces, sometimes marvelous and mysterious, lie within nearly every human soul. Develop, expand and bring out these latent powers.

Make your body splendid, your mind supreme; for then you become your real self, you possess all your attainable powers. And men thus developed possess a capital that can not be financially measured. It is worth infinitely more than money. Within the pages of this volume the pathway leading to these gratifying rewards is clearly described. Adhere to the principles set forth and a munificent harvest of physical, mental and spiritual attainments will surely be yours.

--Bernarr Macfadden

TABLE OF CONTENTS

CHAPTER I: Vitality – What is it?

Vitality first of all means endurance and the ability to live long. It naturally indicates functional and organic vigor. You cannot be vital unless the organs of the body are possessed of at least a normal degree of strength and are performing their functions harmoniously and satisfactorily. To be vital means that you are full of vim and energy, that you possess that enviable characteristic known as vivacity. It means that you are vibrating, pulsating with life in all its most attractive forms. For life, energy, vitality-call it what you wish-in all its normal manifestations, will always be found attractive.

A vital man is at all times thoroughly alive. The forces of life seem to imbue every part of his organism with energy, activity and all characteristics opposed to things inanimate. A vital man is naturally enthusiastic. He can hardly avoid being ambitious. And consequently success, with all its splendid rewards, comes to such a man in abundance. Life to such a man should be resplendent with worthy achievements.

No one belittles the importance of success. Everyone is guided to a large extent by the desire to succeed. When a child toddles off to school the training which he secures there is given for the single purpose of bringing success, but this goal cannot possibly be reached without throbbing vitality. In fact, you are not yourself in every sense unless you possess vitality of this sort. The emotions and instincts that come to one when thoroughly developed, with the vital forces surging within, are decidedly different from those which influence one when lacking in stamina. Many who have grown beyond adult age are still undeveloped, so far as physical condition and vigor is concerned, and this lack of physical development or vitality means immaturity-incompleteness. It means that one is short on manhood or womanhood. This statement, that one's personality, under such circumstances, is not completely brought out, may seem strange to some; but careful reasoning will soon verify its accuracy. Success of the right sort, therefore, depends first of all upon intelligent efforts that are guided day after day, with a view, first of all, of developing the physical organism to the highest possible standard, and maintaining it there.

In other words, it is our first duty to be men, strong and splendid, or women, healthy and perfect, if we are desirous of securing life's most gratifying prizes. Many actually go through life only half alive. They are, to a certain extent, doped by their physical deficiencies. They have been handicapped by a lack of the energy that comes with physical development. They need to be stirred by the regular use of the physical powers of the body. When the body is complete in all of its various parts it is truly a marvelous organism. Throbbing vitality stirs the imagination, gives one courage and capacity, thrills one with the possibilities of life, fires the ambitions. The efforts involved in one's daily duties, be they ever so important, then become mere play. To such a man inactivity is impossible. Every day must be filled with active, interesting duties, and progress in such cases is inevitable. Such a man grows, he improves, he ascends. He becomes a positive dominating force in the world.

Can pulsating, vibrating, vitality of this kind be developed? Can one who lacks enthusiasm and organic vigor obtain these valuable forces? If you have failed up to the present to become a complete man, or a splendid woman, can you achieve these extraordinary rewards in the future? You can rest assured that if the necessary efforts are made a revolution can be wrought in your physical and mental powers. You, too, can feel these throbbing vital forces stirring your every nerve, thrilling your very soul. Go to work, in an intelligent manner, realizing that fundamentally the attainment of these great rewards comes from the development of the highest degree of physical excellence. You must have strength of body. You cannot have too much strength. The more nearly you feel like a strong man the more you can achieve in the desired direction. All successful men are, and have been, men of tremendous energy. Their achievements have been simply the expression of the vitality and nerve force which can no more be repressed than the power of an engine when it has been once liberated. Success is due to the dynamic quality of energy. It is true that physical energy and bodily strength are not sufficient for success in all fields. One must have aptitude for his chosen work. Your energy must be directed in the proper channels, but without this energy and vitality you can accomplish virtually nothing.

Take the one particular characteristic known as vivacity. How we envy those who possess in abundance this great gift! No matter how irregular one's features may be, even though they repel, if a smile shows vivacity associated with a keen, intelligent personality, one cannot be otherwise than attractive. John Bunny, with features rough, unchiseled, ugly, almost uncouth, yet possessed a personality that spread its contagious good humor to millions of people in all quarters of the world who mourned his recent death as that of a personal acquaintance. On the other hand, even though a man or woman possess regular features, the lack of animated expression, of vivacity, causes the person to be regarded as "cold" and "repellent." Speaking in the vernacular, it puts you in the class of the "dead ones." One may say that magnetism and all the desirable qualities that draw others to us are closely associated with the supreme development of the forces of life. No vivacity, then no personality.

The average individual goes through life without living. In other words, he scarcely exists. He has never felt the throbbing exultation of a keen joyous moment. Nor on the other hand has he ever suffered the tortures that are supposed to be associated with the damned, for we must remember that the power to enjoy carries with it a corresponding power to suffer. But we should also remember that the possession of these extremes, the ability to enjoy or to suffer, indicates the attainment of what might be termed the most complete human development. If we wish to find a perfect picture of the phlegmatic temperament, we can study a pig to advantage. And yet there are many human beings incapable of manifesting life-forces equal to those of this humble animal.

But why not be alive, vital, vivacious? Why not be alert, keen, energetic, enthusiastic, ambitious, bubbling over with fiery ardor? The possession of these pulsating, vibratory forces proves that one's physical development has closely approached to perfection. To such vital individuals life opens up opportunities that are almost countless.

But those who have never lived in this "world" of fiery ambitions and throbbing powers, who have never been stirred by the keen, satisfying joys that go with these extraordinary, vital qualities, may ask if these invaluable powers can be developed. Are these stirring, vital forces the possession of favored classes only, or may they be obtained by anyone and everyone? In other words, can they be cultivated or developed? My reply, in nearly all cases, would be in the affirmative. There may be exceptions. There is a limit to the development of the physical force, but health is attainable by the majority. So long as there is life you should be possessed of sufficient vitality to attain a normal degree of health. It really takes more power to run a defective machine than it does to operate one in which all parts are working in harmony, and the same can be said of the body and its parts or organs. Therefore, if you have vitality enough to continue to live even though diseased, rest assured that you have enough to acquire health if you conform to Nature's enactments. And this kind of health usually brings a physical and mental exaltation that is truly beyond description.

It is my purpose in these pages to help the reader to solve the problems associated with the attainment of vitality and health at its best. By following out the suggestions which you will find in this volume, by stimulating the life-forces in connection with the thyroid gland, by straightening and strengthening the spine, by toning up the alimentary canal, and by adopting other suggestions set forth in these pages, you should be insured the attainment of vital vigor really beyond price. Do not be satisfied with an existence. If life is worth anything, it is worth living in every sense of the word. The building up of one's physical assets should be recognized as an imperative duty.

CHAPTER II:
Functional Activity-The Secret of Power

Vitality means normal functioning. When the organs of the body are all performing their duties satisfactorily, you can practically be sure of a plentiful supply of vitality. So it can truly be said that proper functioning is the secret of power.

The most important of all functional processes begins in the stomach. There is where the blood-making process commences, and, since a man is what the blood makes of him, you can realize the tremendous importance of this particular function. If the digestion is carried on properly, and the blood is made rich in those elements that add to life, health and strength, then the functions of the stomach are being properly performed. Strength of this organ, therefore, is absolutely indispensable in vitality building.

This blood-making work is then continued by the small intestines, where a large part of the elements of nourishment essential to life are assimilated, taken up and carried to the portal circulation, thence to the lungs and heart, and finally throughout the entire body. It is absolutely impossible for one to enjoy the possession of a high degree of vitality, or of the general good health upon which vitality depends, unless the intestinal tract is in a healthy and vigorous condition, so that the functions of this particular part of the body-machine may be performed without a flaw. The entire digestive system may be compared to a boiler supplying the energy by which the engine does its work.

Then consider the heart itself. One cannot underestimate the functional importance of this organ. It is commonly regarded as the most vital spot in the body, the very center of life-indeed the poets have made it the seat of love and the emotions in general. If anything, the brain and nervous system should be regarded as the real center of life, but the function of the heart, the marvelous muscle-pump, is so vital and indispensable that the world is accustomed to thinking of it as the organ of first importance. And so it is. Should it cease its efforts for a few moments even, life becomes extinct, and you are no longer an animate being. A strong heart, therefore, is if anything even more important than a strong stomach. But you must remember that the strength of the heart to a large extent depends upon the cooperation of a strong stomach, or at least upon the proper digestion of food. For the muscles and tissues of the heart, like those of all other organs of the body, are fed by the blood, which depends for its life-giving and life-sustaining qualities upon the food, which is first acted upon by the stomach and thus made available for use by the cell structures in all parts of the body. The heart is truly a wonderful organ, the one set of muscles which apparently never rest, but work on night and day, year after year, throughout our entire life.

Furthermore, the part played by the lungs in the maintenance of life and health cannot be underestimated. Impaired functioning of the lungs has an immediate and vital effect upon every other part of the body. It is through this channel that we secure the oxygen, without which the processes of life would terminate almost instantaneously. It is through this channel also that the elimination of carbonic acid gas is accomplished. Without the continuous and thorough elimination of carbonic acid our tissues would become choked up and poisoned in such a way that all cell activity and bodily function would come to an abrupt end. If the lungs are sound and healthy in every respect the supply of oxygen is abundant, and the elimination of carbonic acid, which may be regarded as the "smoke" of the human system, is carried on perfectly. Breathing is only one of the various functions that must be continuously carried on, but it is of such importance as to require special attention in building vitality.

In the work of eliminating impurities and keeping the system clean the kidneys are to be classed with the lungs, although they have to do with poisonous wastes of a different type. Insufficient functioning of the kidneys is not so immediately fatal as the failure of the lungs to do their work, but proper action of the kidneys is none the less important. If the poisons which are normally eradicated from the system in this way are allowed to remain or to accumulate, they poison the body as truly as any external toxic element that could be introduced. Insufficient activity of the kidneys leads to the accumulation of those poisons, bringing on convulsions of the most serious nature, and unless the condition is relieved there will be fatal results. The requirements of health, therefore, demand that the kidneys should be strong and active, and that their functional capacity should be maintained at the highest degree of efficiency.

In supplementing the work of the kidneys and the lungs, the excretory function of the skin is only secondary in importance. The skin has various functions. It is one of our chief organs of sense, the sense of touch being hardly second to those of sight and hearing. It is likewise a wonderful protective structure, and at the same time is a channel of elimination which cannot be ignored with impunity. To interfere with the eliminative function of the skin by absolutely clogging the pores for a period of several hours means death. One may say that we really breathe through the skin.

The importance of all these functions of elimination is vital. Pure blood depends upon the perfect and continuous excretion of the wastes formed in the body through the processes of life, and without keeping the blood pure in this manner the body rapidly becomes poisoned by its own waste products, with the result that health, vitality and even life are lost. Health is entirely a question of pure blood, and, while the blood depends first upon the building material supplied through the digestive system, it also depends equally as much upon functional activity in the matter of elimination.

The liver, which enjoys the distinction of being the largest organ in the body, is designed for the performance of a multiplicity of functions. It not only produces the bile, which has such an important part to play in the work of digestion, but it has a very important work in the changing of foods absorbed into such material as may be assimilated or used by the cells of the various tissues throughout the body. For instance, it is part of the function of the liver to bring about chemical changes in albuminous foods which make it possible for the tissues to assimilate these. It also has much to do with bringing about certain chemical changes in sugar or dextrose. Furthermore, the liver has an important function in connection with the excretion of broken-down bodily tissue, converting this dead matter into a form in which it can be filtered out of the blood by the kidneys. Failure of the liver to perform its work satisfactorily will upset the digestive and functional system, or may lead to an accumulation of uric acid in the body, possibly resulting in rheumatism, gout, neuralgia, disturbances of circulation and other evils. When your liver "goes on strike" you may expect trouble in general. A normal condition of the entire body depends upon perfect and continuous functioning of the liver in cooperation with all the other vital organs. The same may be said of the pancreas, spleen, the thyroid gland and other organs which have a special function to perform. The body is really a combination of all these various parts and functions, and without strength and activity in all of them, simultaneous and harmonious, not one of these interdependent parts could do its work, and the body as a whole would be thrown into a state of disease. Strength of the internal organs is infinitely more important than mere muscular strength, if one could properly make a comparison.

How, therefore, shall we build this internal, functional strength? Can our organs be made to function more satisfactorily? How may we promote their greater activity?

It will be the purpose of the succeeding chapters in this volume to point out how the vital organs may be strengthened and the sum total of one's vitality thereby increased. It is true that internal strength is more important than external muscular strength, but the fact is that they go together. As a general thing, by building muscular strength one is able at the same time to develop internal strength. The influence of exercise in purifying the blood and in promoting activity in all the internal organs really strengthens the "department of the interior" at the same time that it develops the muscles concerned. Muscular stagnation means organic stagnation, to a very large degree. To be thoroughly alive and to enjoy the possession of unlimited vitality it is necessary to be both muscularly and functionally active. The requirements of Nature, or what are more commonly termed the "laws of Nature," in reference to all these bodily functions must be strictly observed, for it is only under such conditions that life and health can be maintained at their best.

The body may be regarded as a machine. Why not make it a strong machine, and as perfect as possible? Its efficiency means everything. If you had an engine, a motorcycle, a sewing machine or a printing press that was a very poor machine, you would like to exchange it for a better one, would you not? You would even spend large sums of money to secure a better machine to take the place of the poor one. But if your body is imperfect, inefficient, weak, rusty and clogged up with grit, dirt and all the waste products due to the "wear" in the bodily structures, you seem nevertheless entirely satisfied. You go on from day to day and from year to year without thinking of the possibility of getting a better physical equipment. But why not consider the body in the same light as any other machine that is of value to you. Your body is the thing that keeps you alive. If it is a poor instrument, then it is more important that you should get a better one than that you should buy a new engine or new printing-press or new sewing-machine. The only difference is, that it is within your power to get a better body machine by building up the one that you have. You can repair it, you can add to its vitality, you can strengthen the functional system, you can make it more perfect and efficient. You can make it a high-power machine that will be of real value in any undertaking that you may wish to carry out. You can make it strong instead of weak, and you can thus enjoy that superabundant vitality without which life is hardly worth the living.

CHAPTER III: The Proper Bodily Posture

The very great value of maintaining the body in a proper position cannot be too strongly emphasized. Man is the only animal that walks erect. He is the only animal in whom old age brings a forward bending of the spine. The hanging head, which is the attitude of hopelessness, and which is caused to a very large extent by the mental attitude that goes with approaching old age, no doubt does a great deal to quicken physical decline.

Therefore it would be wise to remember the very grave importance of a straight, erect spine. Each day of your life should be to a certain extent a fight for the best that there is in life and a struggle to hold the spine as nearly erect as possible. If you are sitting in a chair, sit up straight, head back, chin in. If you are walking or standing, the same rule should apply. The more nearly you can assume the position which is sometimes criticized by the sarcastic statement that "He looks as though he had swallowed a poker," the more nearly you will approximate the ideal position.

As will be shown in the succeeding chapter, it is not necessary to make extraordinary efforts to hold the shoulders back or to arch the chest. The one idea-chin in, down and backward-will accomplish all that is needed. The chest and shoulders will naturally take care of themselves.

Furthermore, it is well to remember that this attitude in itself has a tremendous influence upon both the physical and mental organism. The mind, for instance, is affected to an extraordinary degree by this position. It quickens the reasoning capacity, helps to clear the brain of "cobwebs" and unquestionably adds to one's courage. The man who is afraid hangs his head. He who is void of fear holds his head erect, "looks the world in the face!" There is no question that if a man without fear were to assume the position of fear, with hanging head and shrinking body, he would quickly find himself stirred by the emotions associated with such a posture. He would soon "get scared!" In fact, the attitude of the body has so much to do with one's mental and emotional state that the question of self-confidence or lack of confidence may

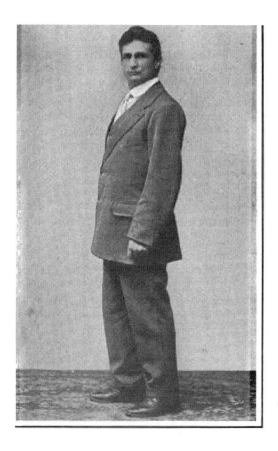

This illustration gives some idea of the proper carriage of the body, with chin in and backward, though in this photograph the head is slightly turned. Struggle for this position when standing or sitting to the fullest extent of your powers throughout every day of your life.

often be decided simply by throwing your head up and back. As will be shown in the succeeding chapter, it is not necessary to make extraordinary efforts to hold the shoulders back or to arch the chest. The one idea-chin in, down and backward-will accomplish all that is needed. The chest and shoulders will naturally take care of themselves.

Furthermore, it is well to remember that this attitude in itself has a tremendous influence upon both the physical and mental organism. The mind, for instance, is affected to an extraordinary degree by this position. It quickens the reasoning capacity, helps to clear the brain of "cobwebs" and unquestionably adds to one's courage. The man who is afraid hangs his head. He who is void of fear holds his head erect, "looks the world in the face!" There is no question that if a man without fear were to assume the position of fear, with hanging head and shrinking body, he would quickly find himself stirred by the emotions associated with such a posture. He would soon "get scared!" In fact, the attitude of the body has so much to do with one's mental and emotional state that the question of self-confidence or lack of confidence may often be decided simply by throwing your head up and back and assuming the general bodily posture that goes with confidence. It not only expresses confidence: it also develops confidence. There is a great truth here that psychologists and those who write "character building" books have not sufficiently understood or emphasized. And when you feel discouraged, the best way to overcome the sense of depression is to "brace up" physically. It will help you to "brace up" mentally. Try it.

Then there are the definite physiological results of maintaining an erect spine. The mechanical arrangement of the spine itself is such that if it is held erect the important nerves that radiate to all parts of the body from this central "bureau" are able more perfectly to perform their functions. Where there is pressure on these nerves there is bound to be imperfect functioning. The affected organ will work lazily, indifferently. In fact, the entire science of the osteopaths and chiropractors is based almost wholly upon the value of spinal stimulation and the remedying of spinal defects.

There is another way in which an erect carriage has a direct physical influence, namely, in maintaining the proper position of the vital organs. When the body is held erect the chest is full, round and somewhat expanded, affording plenty of room for the heart and lungs. This, in itself, is conducive to vitality as compared with the flat-chested attitude. The stomach, liver, spleen, pancreas and intestines all tend to drop or sag below their normal position when the body bends forward. In maintaining an erect position all these organs are drawn upward and held in their natural position, and this means greater vigor and better functioning on the part of each. This particular consideration is of special importance in the case of women. It all goes to show the truly wonderful value of maintaining the spine in a properly erect attitude.

The sitting position usually assumed is far from what it should be in order to insure health. As a rule, we sit humped forward, with a decided bend in the spine, ultimately developing splendid examples of what we call round shoulders. The spine, while sitting, should be held as nearly straight as possible. The position of the head, to a very large extent, determines the general posture of the body. As nearly as possible the chin should be held inward, downward and backward. I will admit that this position is almost impossible when one is using the ordinary type of chair.

An extraordinary effort is required to sit properly in the conventional chair. Furniture of this sort should be made to fit the body in the same way as our clothing does. The back of a chair should be made to fit the backs of those who are to occupy the chair. The chair-back should, at least to a reasonable extent, approximate the normal shape of the spine. If the chair, throughout its entire back, cannot be thus shaped, then it should be cut off even with the waist line of the occupant. Such a low-back chair will usually allow one to sit erect without serious discomfort.

There has been much criticism of American men on the ground that they are inclined to sit down on the small of the back. They slide forward in the chair, with the back bent over and the shoulders humped forward. But the fault really lies with the construction of the chair. The back of a chair does not fit the human back, and the seat is not at the right angle to rest the body.

Why is it that men commonly like to tilt a chair backward on the hind legs? Even when they do not place their feet on a convenient table they are prone to tip the chair back and partly balance it on the hind legs. Why do people instinctively prefer a rocking chair as a source of comfort, even when they do not rock? The fact is that it is not the rocking that makes a rocking chair comfortable, but the position of the seat of the chair, with its downward slope toward the back. The rocking chair is comfortable for just the same reason that the ordinary dining chair is made more comfortable when a man tilts it back upon its hind legs. The reason is that in this position one does not tend to slide forward off the chair, the weight of the body naturally carrying the hips to the back of the chair, where it is supported naturally. In order to avoid the "sliding down the cellar door" character of the conventional chair a change should be made in the incline of the seat similar to that found in the ordinary rocking chair and in the chair when tipped back in the manner I have described.

The photograph which has been reproduced on the following page illustrates the point I wish to make. In this particular instance I have used an ordinary chair to show what can be done to improve the chairs in the ordinary home. Both of the back legs of this chair were sawed off some three or four inches-thus elevating the front part of the chair and lowering the back part, giving the seat an incline toward the rear which more comfortably accommodates the body. This position approximates that of the ordinary swivel desk chair tilted back by business men when they are not leaning forward over their desks. This suggestion can be adopted very easily and cheaply in almost any home, for any ordinary chair treated in this manner will be very greatly improved, and far greater comfort will be experienced as a result of the change. Civilized men and women spend such a very large part of the time in a sitting position that the bodily posture when sitting down is a very great factor in the bodily welfare and health. Special thought and study, therefore, should be given the question of the sitting posture. Unfortunately, this particular subject seems to have been ignored absolutely for hundreds of years in the making of our chairs.

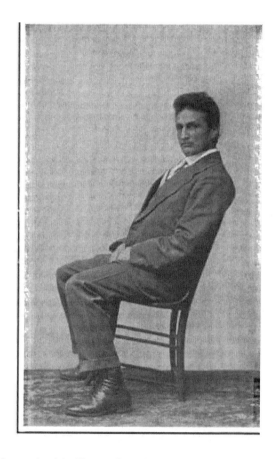

In the chair shown in this illustration the back legs have been sawed off about four inches. This naturally lowers the back, gives it an additional slant and adds very greatly to the comfort of the chair.

It is just as harmful to sit all humped over as it is to stand in such a position. The nervous system cannot be maintained at its best unless the spine is held reasonably erect. Whether sitting or standing, therefore, it is important that you should make a never-ending struggle for a straight spine.

If the back of the chair in which you sit is not properly made then it is better, in most cases, to ignore the back altogether. Sit slightly forward from the back and maintain an erect position, with the chin held in, downward and backward. In this position you should sit well balanced, as it were. The chest should occupy the same relative position as when standing erect. If you will hold the head in the position I have indicated it will help you to keep the chest and back in the right position. As a general thing, it is a much more simple matter to maintain this erect position when sitting, if either one foot, or both feet, are drawn back under the chair. When both feet are stretched out forward upon the floor a person is inclined to sag backward in a partially reclining position upon the chair. By holding one foot underneath the chair in such a manner that you could rise to a standing position, if desired, without lurching forward, you will find it easy to maintain a well balanced and erect posture. If at any time you find yourself slumping forward or slouching in your seat, it is good to stretch your arms high above the head, or to expand the chest and draw your shoulders backward in the position commonly assumed when yawning and stretching. Either of these stretching movements will give you an erect position, and you can maintain this thereafter by keeping the head in the right position-chin inward, downward and backward. These stretching movements will be equally effective for improving the carriage when standing.

The same complaint that I have made against the ordinary chair can be registered with special force against the desks used in the schoolrooms. There is no question that a great deal of spinal curvature in childhood, to say nothing of round shoulders and flat chests, are directly the result of the improper sitting posture in the schools which is enforced upon the children because of the unsuitable character of their seating arrangements. Thus we practically begin life hampered by an unsatisfactory environment, so far as our sitting posture is concerned.

The chair back or the desk chair should fit the human back. It should favor and not hamper one in assuming a normal and straight position of the spine.

When you get up in the morning, exercise yourself a little in straightening the spine, chin in, downward and backward. When you walk to business or when you go about your duties, keep the same thought in mind. Force the head back. Take the exercises which you will find in the next chapter, referring to the thyroid gland, at very frequent intervals during the day.

Remember that in fighting for a straight spine you are fighting for youth and health and life and energy and courage and enthusiasm. You are fighting for everything that is best in life, and you should strive and struggle with all the energy you possess to win the rewards associated therewith.

Each day of your life will bring difficulties, worries. Life at its best is not a bed of roses. All these various influences are inclined to make you hang your head. You may have moments when you are hopeless, when life seems forbidding and cheerless. Fight against such inclinations with all the power you possess. Struggle against such discouragements with all your might and main, not only through your mental attitude but through your determination to maintain an erect spine. Hold your head up and look the world in the face.

Don't shirk your duty. Don't deviate from the path along which your best impulses and highest ideals would lead you. Life is worth while. It is filled with glorious opportunities. Reach out and grasp them as they come up. Hold your head up and be a man or a woman to the fullest extent of your abilities.

CHAPTER IV:
Stimulating the Source of Stamina and Vitality

This is an age of short cuts. Any devious routes to the accomplishment of an object should be avoided. If you want vitality, and the vivacity, energy and enthusiasm with which it is associated, you naturally search for a method which will bring certain and quick improvements. The reasonableness and general prevalence of this demand was in my mind when I began experimentation with a view to discovering a method for stimulating what I term the source of vital power.

Scientific men while delving into the marvelous secrets of physiology, have learned that the thyroid gland in some peculiar manner possesses an extraordinary influence upon vital stamina and virility. This mysterious gland is located in front of the neck, about half way between the so-called "Adam's apple" and the top of the sternum or breast-bone, where it adheres to each side of the front of the trachea, or windpipe, in a flattened form, something like the wings of a butterfly, with a connecting "isthmus." It is a "ductless" gland, its secretions apparently being taken up by absorption into the lymph, and from that into the blood.

While the functions of this little organ are not yet very clearly understood, there is nothing more definitely known than its tremendous importance in the bodily economy. Without it there can be no such thing as healthy development. Thyroid deficiency in children gives rise to a form of idiocy, bodily malformation and degeneracy known as cretinism, while in adult life it is associated with a similar disorder known as myxedema. Goiter is the most common disorder of the thyroid gland; though not very serious in minor cases, it is capable of becoming very dangerous, assuming such malignant forms as exophthalmic goiter, which is marked by palpitation of the heart, nervous symptoms and protrusion of the eyes.

It is thought by some authorities that the thyroid gland has to do with the control of the excretion of the waste products from nitrogenous foods, for it has been found that a meat diet or a high-proteid diet is extremely harmful in disorders of this organ. It has been found that dogs fed on meat after the thyroid gland has been removed invariably die in a few days, but that they can be kept alive for a long time if fed on a diet very low in proteids. It is found as a rule that those suffering from thyroid troubles do very well on a milk diet.

Some students of the subject conclude that the function of the thyroid gland is to destroy poisonous products formed by the decomposition of proteid food substances. It is believed by others that it also has a defensive action against other poisons in the body, including alcohol and poisonous drugs. In other words, it is thought to have an "antitoxic" action. It has also been held that this organ has much to do with the supply of iodine in the system, being particularly affected by the lack of iodine in the food. Again, it is said that when the thyroid gland has degenerated there ensues a condition of auto-intoxication, followed by a degeneration of other organs which destroy and eliminate poisons in the blood. It is claimed that in many cases of thyroid deficiency, as in cretinism, good results have been obtained by the use of thyroid extract, thus supplying the body with the secretion which normally should have been obtained from this gland.

But, whatever may be the function of this remarkable little organ, the fact remains that it is of tremendous importance to health, being undeniably endowed with extraordinary influence on virility, physical strength and mental vigor. Now these facts were in mind when I commenced the experiments which, as I have said, led to the discovery of a method of stimulating the vital forces of the body. The problem seemed simple in some respects. If the thyroid gland has such a definite effect upon bodily health, the query as to how it can be strengthened and stimulated to perform its work more satisfactorily, assumed unusual importance and I was strongly moved to discover the answer. The problem, however, was not by any means an easy one. A long time elapsed before a satisfactory solution presented itself. The first thought that naturally occurs to one when endeavoring to stimulate the activities of any part of the body is to find some means of increasing the circulation to that part. Ordinary massage will usually accomplish this purpose to a limited degree, though massage to my

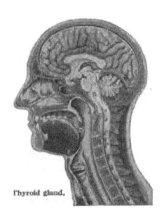

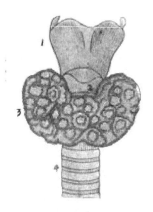

Thyroid gland.
At the right, thyroid gland, larynx and trachea (windpipe) of one-year old child.

1. Larynx.
2. Cricold Cartilage.
3. Thyroid gland.
4. Trachea.

mind is a superficial agent in many cases. It will increase local circulation, but it does not facilitate tissue changes to the same extent as exercise which directly affects the structures concerned, or the mechanical movements of the parts themselves that are brought about through active use of them in some way. I have known of cases in which pressure and massage applied to the region of the thyroid gland have been followed by harmful effects, such as fainting, and certainly no one with a weak heart should attempt to stimulate this organ in this manner. Therefore, in endeavoring to find a satisfactory means of stimulating this important gland, I did not give massage serious thought. And I might as well say that I finally "stumbled" upon the important truth which is the basis of the method that I am presenting.

For many years I have been a student of vocal culture, having taken up the study of this art chiefly as a recreation, with no thought of ever publicly using any ability I might acquire, though I might mention that the additional vocal strength obtained as a result of this training assisted me greatly in public speaking. While giving my attention to this particular study, I was greatly impressed by the extreme importance of maintaining an erect spine, holding the chin down, inward and backward, and keeping the shoulders back and the chest expanded. I found, however, like many others who become "slack" in bodily posture, that a considerable effort was required to maintain a proper position at all times. I therefore began a series of special exercises intended really to force myself to assume a properly erect position. While experimenting with these exercises for the purpose mentioned, I noted a marked effect upon my general vital vigor. Not only was this made apparent by an increase in physical strength and stamina, but it was marked in an equal degree by additional mental energy and capacity. My mind was clearer, and I could surmount difficulties presented in business enterprises in which I was interested with far more ease than before. I could make decisions more easily and quickly. In addition, a decided gain in weight was noted-not by any means in the form of mere fatty tissue, but of firm, substantial flesh. These very pleasing results induced me to go more carefully into the causes underlying this remarkable improvement. I carried on an

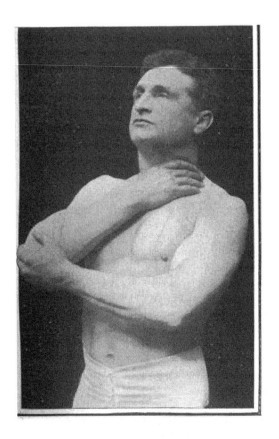

EXERCISE 1.
Place the right open palm over the lower portion of the neck
covering the thyroid gland and press slightly. If one is especially
vigorous, the pressure can be considerably increased by adding
the strength of the left arm as illustrated.

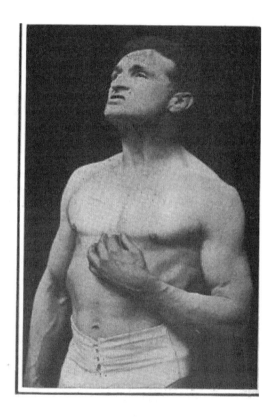

EXERCISE 2.
Bring the chin far upward, then stretch the platysma myoides
muscle lying immediately in front of the neck, and spreading out
across the upper part of the chest; repeat until it is fatigued.

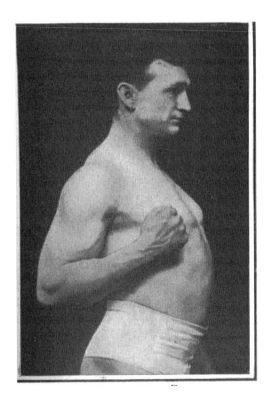

EXERCISE 3

Move chin inward, slightly downward and as far backward as possible. This movement is so slight that it can be used at any time, walking, sitting, or standing, even while conversing with a friend, as it will hardly be noticed. Make the effort as vigorous as possible each time the head is moved backward. Always be sure the abdomen is expanded while making these movements.

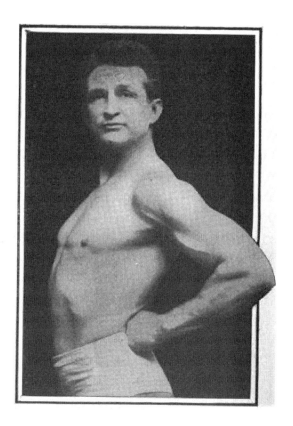

EXERCISE 4.

A movement very similar to the preceding, though the head is turned far to the side as will be noted. Vary the movement by turning to the right or to the left side. This movement and the preceding one illustrated represent two of the most important features of thyroid stimulation. They should be used at frequent intervals throughout every day.

elaborate series of careful experiments with a view to proving the conclusions to which I had come in the course of these exercises. It was quite apparent that a full development of the back part of the upper spine was necessary in order to maintain the strength essential to extreme vigor and vitality. And it became quite plain to me that this development could not be achieved without stimulating to an unusual degree the thyroid gland. Reasoning along this line, I called to mind the appearance of various animals noted for their great strength and there I found my conclusions verified with remarkable emphasis. The arched neck of the stallion, the huge development of the back of the neck of the domestic bull, the same character in even more pronounced form in the case of the bull buffalo and the musk-ox, and in varying degrees in other animals conspicuous for their vitality and energy-all this seemed to indicate that I was on the verge of a remarkable discovery. When you think of a fiery steed, in every instance you bring to mind the arched appearance of the neck. The tight reins that are sometimes used to give a horse a pleasing appearance, are based upon the same ideal, showing a more or less subconscious recognition of the idea that this particular development is associated with tremendous animal vigor.

After giving consideration to various methods that could be used for the purpose of stimulating this little organ, the thyroid gland, I finally concluded as the result of prolonged experimentation that the exercises illustrated in this chapter can most thoroughly be depended upon for producing results. All movements here described have proved effective in imparting to the neck a full, arched, well developed appearance, but I have given especial attention to the active use of the muscles on the back of the neck. Nearly every movement which to a certain extent develops these muscles is inclined to stimulate the thyroid gland. The more special movements for this purpose are indicated in the various illustrations accompanying this chapter. This development of the back of the neck always indicates great vitality, because definite proof is thereby given that the spine is unusually strong and is maintained in a position favorable to the functioning of all the organs of the body. Many of the movements illustrated are but slight in character, but they

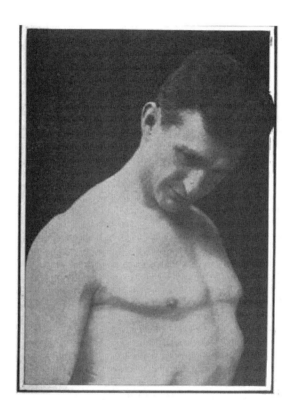

EXERCISE 5.
Bring the chin vigorously far downward on the chest with
muscles tightly tensed and with head held far downward, twist far
to the right then far to the left.

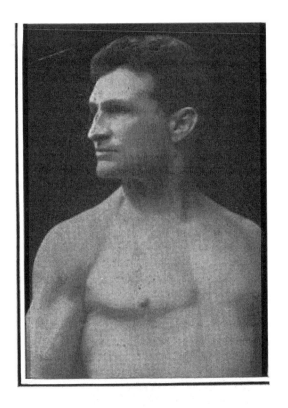

EXERCISE 6.
Reach outward far to the side with your chin, endeavoring as
nearly as possible to touch the right shoulder with it. Repeat the
movement, stretching far outward and endeavoring to touch the
left shoulder with the chin.

are the more adaptable because of this. No matter where you may be, whether walking along the street, conversing with a friend, or sitting at a desk, they can be practiced quietly without attracting attention. Furthermore, it is absolutely essential that an erect position of the spine be kept in mind continually. You should begin every morning to hold the spine straight and erect, and each day should represent an increment of success in the struggle finally to maintain involuntarily this position of the body. On arising in the morning, practice some of the exercises illustrated in this chapter for stimulating the thyroid gland, being careful to perform them just as instructed in each illustration. Whenever you are unoccupied during the day, it is a good plan to practice these movements occasionally, as they will assist you materially in maintaining the spine in that erect position which I found so important at the beginning of my vocal studies.

The most important movement is to bring the chin downward, inward, and backward as far as possible, endeavoring to arch as much as you can the back of the neck. You may have to practice a long while before you notice an outline that will in any way resemble an arch in the back of your neck, but all this work you can be assured will be of decided benefit to you. And, whether or not you attain the desired arch, you can be assured of benefits that will be worth all your efforts. When you make these movements properly, there is no necessity for trying to bring the chest out or the shoulders far back. The simple movements of the neck alone as described, if properly performed, will fulfill all requirements. For these movements tend mechanically to raise and arch the chest and to throw the shoulders far backward. Remember also the necessity, when taking these movements, of keeping the abdominal region expanded as fully as possible. Do not draw in the waist line. The importance of this admonition cannot be too strongly emphasized. If you maintain a full abdomen, thyroid-stimulating movements seem to tone up, increase in size, and strengthen all the vital organs lying in the gastric region.

In further proof of the value of the exercises described in this work as a means of building unusual vital vigor, note the remarkable stamina and virility of men possessing an unusual development of the neck.

Where the neck is broad and well filled out at the back, you can depend absolutely upon the possession of great vital vigor. It is quite plain, therefore, that by merely adopting some method of developing this part of the spine you will have accomplished a great deal towards obtaining a high degree of vital stamina. Some of the strongest men in the world can be found among professional wrestlers. Many of those following this profession retain their athletic ability a great many years beyond the athletic life of men in other branches of sport. In fact, champion wrestlers sometimes retain their championship honors for a score of years beyond the age at which champion boxers and runners retire. It is a well known fact that wrestling requires extraordinary strength of the upper spine. Some of the most strenuous wrestling holds use the muscles of the upper back and neck in a very vigorous and violent manner. Consequently wrestlers are noted for what are often termed bull necks, thus plainly indicating the exceptional degree of vital vigor which they possess.

Accordingly it is well to remember in connection with these exercises that many movements which assist in the development of the neck muscles also serve to stimulate the activities of the thyroid gland. You cannot go through the process of training for a wrestling match without stimulating this organ to an exceptional degree. Therefore, in following the suggestions which are given in this chapter, you are securing the full benefit of a vitality-stimulating process that ordinarily can be obtained only by going through a prolonged course of wrestling. There is no necessity for you to develop a "bull neck," but you should make the most strenuous efforts to acquire a sufficient development of the back of the neck to give it an arched appearance. The more nearly you can approximate a development of this character, the more vital will you become. And along with this superior power will come a similar improvement in every other capacity, mental as well as physical.

That there may be no mistake, let me reiterate: That the spine must be held erect at all times when sitting or standing. That frequently during the day when sitting or standing the chin should be brought down and in with a backward movement, the head being turned at times far either to the right or left side, with a vigorous twist of the strongly tensed muscles.

That on every occasion when this movement is made, the abdomen must be fully expanded-not held in or drawn upward.

That great emphasis must be given to the importance of bringing the chin slowly but vigorously downward against the chest before the inward and backward movement is begun. This insures a proper stimulation of the thyroid gland.

CHAPTER V: Stimulating, Straightening and Strengthening the Spine

The human spine bears the same relation to the body as a whole as the trunk of a tree does to the rest of the tree. If the trunk is strong the entire tree is sturdy and vigorous. If the spine is strong the body as a whole possesses a similar degree of strength. Therefore, the necessity for a strong spine is readily apparent.

This strength is necessary not only because the spine is what may be termed the foundation for our entire physical structure but also because therein are located the nerves that radiate to each organ and every minute part of the body. These spinal nerves control the functional processes of all our bodily tissues and structures. If the spine possesses a proper degree of strength, if the bony structure is properly proportioned, and if the alignment of all the vertebrae is everything that can be desired, you are then practically assured of the pulsating vitality which is a part of superb health.

It is an interesting fact that the spine is the central and fundamental structure of all the higher organisms on this earth. In the course of the evolution of life on this planet there developed from the very simplest forms of animal organisms two different higher forms of life--on the one hand the vertebrate animals, possessing an internal skeleton, and on the other hand the insects, clams, crustaceans and other creatures that have their skeletons on the outside, as one may say, in the form of shells. The legs of an insect, for instance, are small tubes with the muscles inside. The limbs of vertebrate animals, on the other hand, have the muscle outside the bone. Invertebrates commonly have the main nerve trunk in front, or underneath, instead of at the back, and likewise often have their brains in their abdomens. Some of them, such as the grasshopper, even hear with their abdomens. But all vertebrata have the great nerve trunk at the back, contained in the spine and with a bulb on the front or upper end constituting the brain. In fact, a vertebrate animal is primarily a living spine, and all other parts of the body are in the nature of appendages. The limbs, for instance, and in the higher animals the ribs and other parts of the skeleton, are simply attached to the spine, or are offshoots from it. In the fishes these limbs take the shape of fins. In the higher developments of life they assume the form of legs.

All the higher animals, as we know, have evolved from the fishes and reptiles, and all in common possess a spine which in its fundamental characteristics is very much the same now as when it was first evolved. In other words, the spine is a bodily structure as old as the rock-ribbed hills. It has stood the test of time, and therefore must be regarded as the most highly perfected mechanical structure in the body. Its strength combined with its flexibility and its perfect adjustment as a container for the central nervous system, makes it perhaps the most wonderful structure in the body outside of the brain and the spinal cord itself. While other organs and features of the body have been changed and modified to such an extent in the various species which have been evolved that they can hardly be recognized as having a common origin, yet the spine has remained substantially the same. It is true that the spine has been shortened in many species as the result of the loss of the tail, but this means only the dropping off of a part of it and does not greatly alter its fundamental character.

The human spine, however, differs from that of other animals in respect to its suitability for the erect posture. Man is the only animal in the world who can straighten his body and stand perfectly erect. Even the anthropoid apes when standing on their feet assume a somewhat oblique position. The vertebral column in animal life was first developed on the horizontal plane, and so, naturally, when man was evolved and adopted the erect position, certain modifications of the spine were necessary. A new strain developed on the vertebral column which was due to the new position, and so there came about certain changes in its structure. For one thing the spine became less flexible and gained in stability, especially in the lower sections. The sacrum, for instance, is created by the fusing together of several vertebrae into one bone for the sake of greater strength and stability. The sacrum in man is much broader than in animals, for it must supply solidity and strength to the lower part of the spine, thus adapting it to the vertical position, and in the same way the lower vertebrae generally are

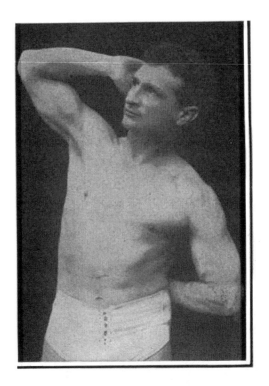

EXERCISE 7.
Move the head far over to the left. Now place the palm of the right hand against the side of the head and press against the head as it is moved from far to the right to far to the left. Continue until slightly fatigued, and then take the same exercise reversing the position by using the left hand against the head instead of the right.

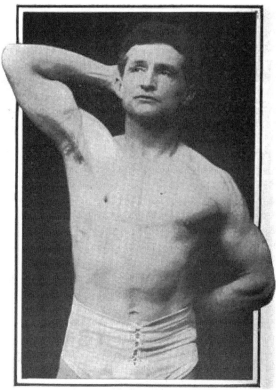

EXERCISE 8.

EXERCISE 8.
Place the right hand behind the head. Now pressing against the head with the right hand, bring the head from far forward to far backward. Continue until tired and vary the movement by using at times the left hand instead of the right.

comparatively broader and heavier, gradually decreasing in size and tapering toward the top of the spine like the trunk of a tree.

This particular feature of the human backbone is worthy of special consideration because it is the upper section of the spine, in which the vertebrae are smaller and tapering, that weakness is most likely to exist. It is in this upper section of the spine that strength is most needed in order to preserve it in perfect alignment, and keep the body properly erect. And it is for this reason, as the reader will see, that exercises affecting the upper parts of the spine are most important. Therefore I have given them special attention.

The curves in the human spine are characteristic, illustrating in another way the modification of the vertebral column that has been made necessary by the erect position. The new-born baby has a backbone that is almost straight, and in this respect it bears a strong resemblance to that of many of the lower animals. The typical human curves, however, begin to take form as soon as the child learns to sit up, and they become more marked as he learns to walk and run. These curves are essential to maintaining the balance of the body in the erect position.

There are really three curves in the human backbone, the cervical curve being convex, the dorsal concave, and the lumbar convex, when each is regarded from the forward aspect. If we consider the sacrum and coccyx, there is really a fourth curve, this being concave, although in animals generally the coccyx curves backwards and is extended to form the tail. In some of the lower animals the spine is nearly straight, while in some cases it virtually forms a complete arch from one end to the other.

These curves of the spine are generally more marked in the civilized white races than among the black and savage races, and as a rule they are more pronounced among women than among men. For instance, in comparing the sexes we find that in a woman the lumbar curve is more marked and extends slightly higher than in a man, and that the broad sacrum characteristic of the human race is even wider, being thus

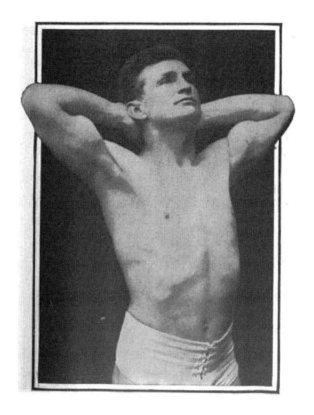

EXERCISE 9.
Interlace the fingers of both hands behind the head. Now with the head far forward, press against the head as it is moved far backward to the position illustrated above. Continue the movement until fatigued.

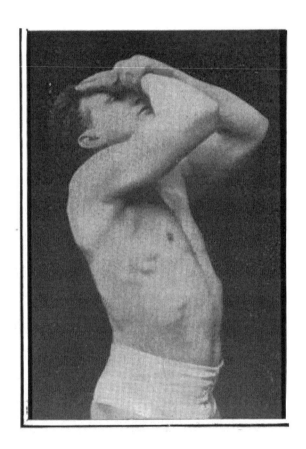

EXERCISE 10.

Place the palm of the left hand across the forehead with the head far back as shown in the illustration, clasping the left wrist with the right hand. Now bring the head far forward, resisting the movement vigorously with the strength of both arms. Continue until tired.

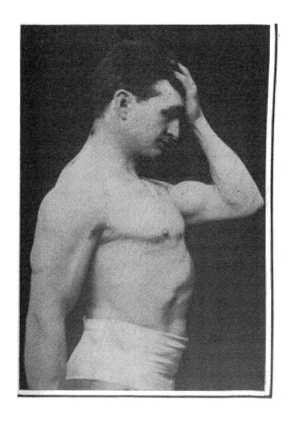

EXERCISE 11.

Place the open palm of the left hand on the forehead. Now while pressing vigorously against the movement, bring the head from far backward to far forward. Continue until fatigued and vary the exercise by using the right hand instead of the left.

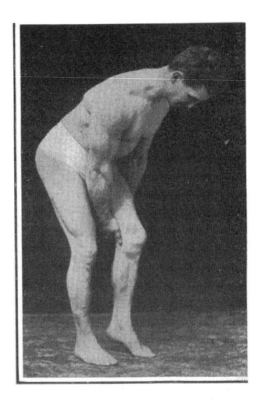

EXERCISE 12.

Interlace fingers behind the left leg just above the knee. Now while slightly resisting the movement with the leg lift upward vigorously. Continue the movement until a slight feeling of fatigue is produced. In addition to its value as a stimulant to the nerve centers this movement is especially recommended for strengthening and developing what is known as "the small of the back." It should be varied by interlacing fingers behind the right leg instead of the left.

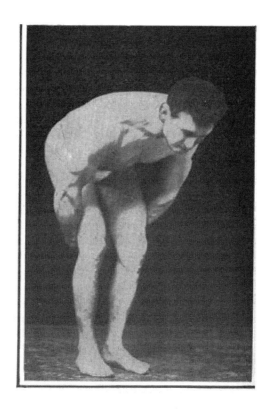

EXERCISE 13.
Hook the fingers of the right and left hands together at the back of
both legs a little above the knee as shown in the illustration. Now
make a vigorous lift upward. Relax and repeat until a definite
sensation of fatigue is produced.

adapted to the broader hips and wider pelvic cavity of the child-bearing sex.

Now, the maintenance of a strong and erect spine, and especially of the normal curves of youth is most important. With the weakness of advancing age the curves, particularly in the upper part of the spine, tend to become more pronounced. The more accentuated these curves are the greater is the weakness of the spine and of the muscles of the back that is indicated. It is said that a man is as old as his spine, since the deterioration of the spine means the loss of elasticity and supporting power in the disk-like cartilages between the vertebrae, and also the loss of strength in the muscles and ligaments of the back which tend to hold the spinal vertebrae in place. It is usually found that vigorous old men who are mentally and physically active at eighty or ninety years are those who have maintained an erect bearing until late in life, who have kept their spines straight and strong instead of allowing them to bend over and double up. In other words, the deterioration of the spine means a general loss of bodily vigor and a decline in the nervous energy or vitality.

With the flattening down of the cushiony disks or cartilages between the vertebrae, and also with the dislocation even in the slightest degree of these vertebrae, there is brought about more or less interference with the free action of the spinal cord itself and of the spinal nerves. The pinching of these nerves naturally interferes with the supply of energy to the organs controlled by them, and causes more or less serious derangement of the bodily functions. If one can keep his spine straight and strong the central nervous system will likewise be healthy and vigorous, and all organs will be supplied with a normal amount of energy and vitality.

The special exercises for the spine which I have recommended for years have the general effect not only of maintaining the proper alignment of the vertebrae and thus promoting the health and welfare of the central nervous system, but also of strongly stimulating the nervous system, and thus toning up the entire bodily organism. All movements of the spine, whether of a twisting or bending character, naturally influence the spinal cord and the spinal nerves in a mechanical way. The result is something akin to a massage of these nerve structures, and in this way, as I have long contended, it is possible directly to stimulate the source of energy and vitality. I am convinced for this reason that muscular exercise for the back is infinitely more important than for any other part of the body, important as it is for all parts. If one has only very little time each day to devote to exercise, then it would pay him best to give that time to movements which will strengthen and stimulate the spine.

The various movements that I am presenting in this chapter have been devised especially to accompany the hot-water regimen that will be described in the following chapter. They are intended not only to add to the strength of the backbone itself, but have been devised with a view to stimulating to an unusual degree the nerve centers located in the spine. As I have already said, the spinal nerves control the functions of all the vital organs, and when the activity of these organs is stimulated not only through increased nerve force but also by the increased supply of blood that will result from the hot water-drinking regimen referred to, then indeed will we have a combination of stimulating forces which will bring about vital changes, in very many cases, little short of astounding in character.

Each of these exercises should be taken until a feeling of fatigue has been noticed, after which you may rest a few moments, breathing fully and deeply with expanded abdomen. You should then be ready to begin the next exercise. There is little danger of soreness from taking these movements when they are combined with hot water-drinking, as recommended in Chapter VI, The water seems to cleanse the tissues of the waste products which ordinarily cause soreness when one begins the practice of exercises to which one is not accustomed. If one possesses unusual vigor, then to the exercises illustrated in this chapter may be added those movements appearing in the following chapter. All of the exercises given in this chapter are designed exclusively for the stimulation of the spine and nerve centers. Those illustrated in the next chapter are intended chiefly to accelerate the circulation throughout the chest, arms, legs and body as a whole, for when going through a treatment of this character it is naturally advisable for one to arouse the activity of all the functions associated with tissue changes throughout all parts of the body.

Although these exercises have not been devised especially for corrective purposes in cases of spinal curvature, yet they will be of exceptional value in all such cases, or at least, where there is no radical mechanical deformity of the vertebral column. Curvatures may be prevented in all cases, or may be decreased, or even reduced entirely by exercise of this type. Incidentally the practice of exercises for improving the spine and giving one the proper erect carriage has a very marked effect upon the chest. An erect position always means expanded chest walls, with plenty of room for the free activity of the heart and lungs.

CHAPTER VI:
Cleansing and Stimulating the Alimentary Canal

The alimentary canal has been rightly termed the human fire-box. It is there that the energy is created which runs the human machine. The importance of cleanliness in this part of the physical organism cannot be too greatly emphasized. Nearly all diseases have their beginning in the stomach or some other part of the alimentary canal. Defective digestion and imperfect assimilation represent the beginning of many incurable and deadly diseases.

In seeking methods for building unusual vigor and vitality, one of the first requirements is definite information on the care of the alimentary canal. Mere regularity of the bowels does not in all cases indicate a healthy condition of the stomach and bowels. A movement in order to be of the right sort should be so thorough that it leaves one with a feeling of emptiness and cleanliness. In other words, you should feel that the colon has been evacuated thoroughly. Many who have regular bowel movements do not have this satisfying sensation afterwards. When the movement is satisfactory in every way little or no straining is necessary. The colon simply empties itself thoroughly, and the evacuation is then complete. However, few have movements of the bowels that are satisfactory to this extent. There should be at least one bowel movement of this kind each day. Two movements of this character would be better, but one is sufficient if thorough.

Do not acquire the idea that the bowels must move at a certain time each day with unintermitted regularity, for they are subject to the same extent as the appetite to what might be termed idiosyncrasies, according to environment and other influences. For instance, you are not always hungry at meal-time. Occasionally you eat very little or skip one or more meals, and it would be a serious mistake to goad your appetite with some stimulant or to eat a meal without an appetite. One can hardly say that to force a bowel movement when its necessity is not naturally indicated is as harmful as to eat a meal when it is not craved, but unquestionably it is of advantage to have the bowels move of their own accord, as the result of a natural impulse. Movements that do not come through the call of an instinct for relief are rarely satisfactory, and, though we strongly emphasize the necessity of regularity of the bowels, it is not absolutely necessary that this call should come at a certain time during each day; and though it is undoubtedly of some advantage if such is the case, yet so long as there is one evacuation each day of the satisfactory sort described, you can be assured that your alimentary canal is in a normal and healthy condition.

However, should the bowels fail to move at the regular time this need not cause concern if you are feeling "up to the mark," and there are no other symptoms that would indicate possible trouble. I mention this alimentary peculiarity to enable my readers to avoid the slavish idea that it is impossible to be in health unless the bowels move at certain times with clock-like regularity.

Naturally when the contents of the alimentary canal are allowed to accumulate for a considerable period and there is sluggishness throughout the various parts of the small and large intestines, poisons of all kinds are generated and absorbed into the circulation, thus creating conditions ranging all the way from a feeling of lethargy to a condition of weakness and disease that confines one to an invalid's bed. Regardless of the attention that you may give to the other information in this book, it is extremely important that you should realize the necessity for active elimination.

It is necessary in the maintenance of alimentary health to avoid a slavish adherence to the theory of definitely regular movements of the bowels and still not to make the mistake of allowing them to become chronically sluggish or irregular. As a rule you should depend upon having regular movements each day, though if occasionally a day is missed you should not allow this deviation to worry you.

Recognizing as I do the great importance of a healthy alimentary canal I have given a vast amount of attention to the various methods which have been suggested from time to time by students of natural healing for assisting to regulate the functional processes of this important part of our organism. The flushing of the lower bowel for instance has been

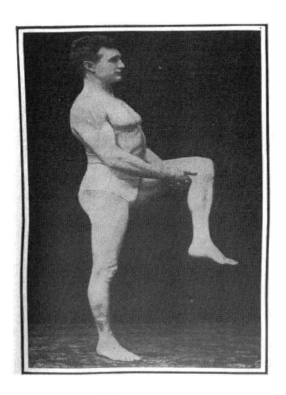

EXERCISE 14.

Stand erect, spine rigid and straight as possible., Bring the left leg upward, bending the knee and grasping the leg almost under the knee as shown. Now lift the leg as high as possible by merely bending the arms at the elbow. This is an unusually valuable exercise for developing the biceps and other muscles of the upper arm The movement should be continued until fatigue ensues. The leg should be varied from left to right at different times when the exercise is taken.

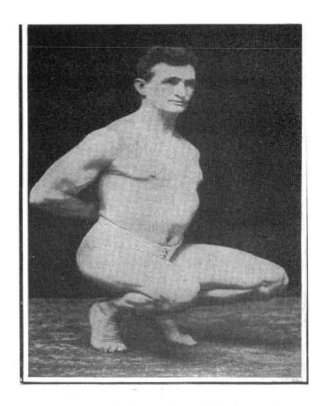

EXERCISE 15.

Stand erect, bend the knees, lowering the body to the crouching position illustrated above. Rise and repeat until a distinct feeling of fatigue is noticed. On each occasion when rising to an erect position, be sure to "snap" the knees backward with a slight "jerk" at the end of the movement. This little movement seems to very greatly stimulate the circulation and materially increase the number of times you can perform the exercise.

widely recommended, and it is unquestionably of value in some cases. However, it cleanses only the lower part of the alimentary canal, that is to say, the colon. It assists the small intestines no doubt by giving their contents free access to the colon, but yet this aid cannot directly affect them. If you have in view the cleansing of the entire alimentary canal from stomach to rectum, the enema is often of indifferent value. The use of various laxative foods can be recommended in most instances, though even these sometimes fail to bring about satisfying results, and then again there are cases where they provide a remedy for only a short period, after which the bowels resume their old state of chronic torpidity. Naturally we cannot consider cathartics of any kind, notwithstanding their power to produce temporary results. In all cases the after effects of their use are seriously destructive to the delicate nerves controlling the alimentary canal and its functions in general. Cathartics invariably make the real condition more obstinate and serious.

It is well to remember that the real cause of constipation in virtually every instance, is the want of vital vigor of the structures and tissues involved. Digestion, though to a certain extent a chemical process, is very largely mechanical. The muscles of the stomach "churn" the food in the beginning of the digestive process, after which the circulatory muscle fibers of the small intestines continue the work. If these muscles are lacking in tone, if they are relaxed, prolapsed and weak, then they cannot properly perform their functions. In attempting to strengthen this important part of the bodily organism the necessity for increasing the vigor of the muscular tissues must invariably be definitely recognized. Strong muscles for carrying on the work required of these blood-making organs are of far more importance than strength of the external muscles. For this reason when the system is toned up by any means a beneficial change in the alimentary functions and excretions will always be noted.

During a careful study extending over at least a quarter of a century of all health-building methods, I have acquainted myself with numerous theories and remedies which have been applied in accelerating alimentary activity. I am, in this chapter, presenting a new system or combination of means for strengthening and stimulating the alimentary functions which experience has proved to be of extraordinary value. This method has the advantage of directly affecting the organs involved, and results can be obtained speedily in virtually every instance.

This system of alimentary stimulation can be roughly described as a combination of hot-water-drinking and a nerve-center-stimulating process. The best time for giving this method a thorough trial is immediately upon arising in the morning. It should not be attempted at any other time of the day, for it is especially important that the stomach should be free of any recently ingested food.

All that is required to carry out this treatment is one or two quarts of boiling water, a minute quantity of salt, and a cup that will hold from one-half a pint to one pint of water. The second phase of this treatment is exercise and comprises the series of movements illustrated in this work. Wherever possible these nerve-stimulating exercises should be taken out-of-doors or before an open window. If the weather is cold, you should wear enough clothing to maintain a satisfactory degree of warmth; if the weather is warm, the less clothing worn the better. If the skin is especially inactive, or if it is suffering from a disease in which the eliminating process ordinarily accelerated by a Russian or Turkish bath is of value, then wear heavy warm clothing while taking the treatment. A thick sweater is advantageous under such circumstances. A profuse perspiration will result, indicating a purifying process that is of special value when the system needs to be cleansed of the accumulated poisons which are the direct cause of nearly all diseases.

If you are capable of taking about two quarts of water in the course of the exercise then each cup should contain nearly a pint, but if you cannot drink over one quart each cup should contain not more than half a pint.

Before beginning the nerve-stimulating exercise drink the first cup of hot water, putting a pinch of salt in the bottom of the cup to take away the flat taste of the hot water. Pour the cup half full of boiling water and

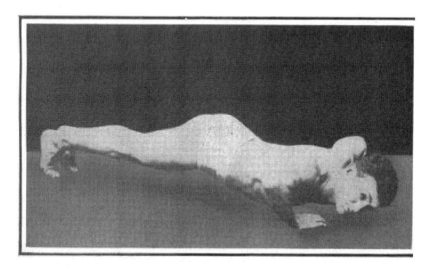

Exercise 16.
Lie prone on the floor, face downward. Place the open hands near the chest, the elbow extended far out at the sides. Raise body by straightening the arms. This exercise and the one which follow (No. 17) are especially valuable for general chest stimulation.

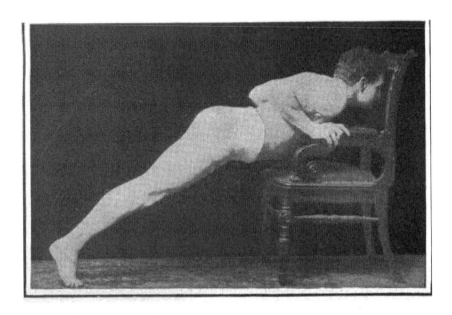

Exercise 17,
The body erect, eblows close to the sides, raise the body by
straightening the arms. A railing, table, chair, the foot of a bed or
anything that will support the body in this position can be used for this
exercise.

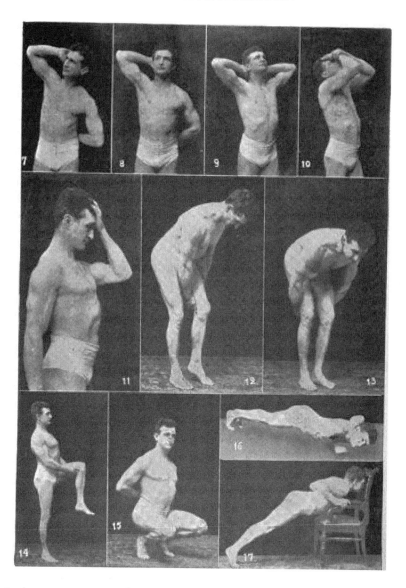

A chart or resume of Exercises 7 to 17, described In the chapters on The Spine and The Alimentary Canal.

then add cold water until it is sufficiently cool to be rapidly swallowed. Drink the water as hot as possible without sipping it. Now take exercises 11, 12 and 14. Continue each one of these movements until a feeling of fatigue is noticed, after which you are ready for a second cup of hot water.

Don't hurry. Don't continue any movement to exhaustion, though a feeling of local fatigue in the particular muscles concerned is desirable. This feeling, however, should entirely disappear after a rest of one or two minutes.

After the second cup of hot water you are ready for exercises 13, 7 and 8, whereupon you may take a third cup of hot water. You may then take exercises 15, 16 and 9, followed by another cup of hot water, and then exercises 17, 6 and 10, and so on. While this is suggested as a general plan, it is not imperative that this order be followed strictly, for your individual requirements might be better suited by minor variations; for instance, by two or four exercises between the intervals of hot-water-drinking.

If you find your capacity is unequal to the quantity of hot water suggested, then simply take as much as you can without inconvenience or discomfort. Each day, however, while following this method you will find your hot-water-drinking capacity will increase, though as a rule, a person of average weight and height can take from one to two quarts without serious inconvenience. The hot-water drinking together with the exercise will naturally very greatly increase the pulse, and where there is heart disease or any weakness of the heart this treatment must be taken with unusual care. In virtually every case this method will materially increase the strength of a weak heart, though there is naturally the possibility of strain, and the treatment should be adapted to your strength in the beginning and very gradually increased week by week.

Temporary attacks of constipation, where severe enough to need attention, can usually be ready for exercises 13, 7 and 8, whereupon you may take a third cup of hot water. You may then take exercises 15, 16 and 9, followed by another cup of hot water, and then exercises 17, 6 and 10, and so on.

While this is suggested as a general plan, it is not imperative that this order be followed strictly, for your individual requirements might be better suited by minor variations; for instance, by two or four exercises between the intervals of hot-water-drinking.

Temporary attacks of constipation, where severe enough to need attention, can usually be quickly remedied by this hot-water drinking, nerve-stimulating method. Usually, if there is need for a movement of the bowels an instinctive and compelling desire will appear while taking the treatment or very shortly thereafter. If, however, you feel there is a necessity for such a movement and it does not appear, you can rest assured that the treatment has brought about sufficient benefit to excite the activity of the organs involved and that the desire will come later. In some very obstinate cases of constipation, or in serious temporary attacks of this difficulty, where a movement of the bowels is desired quickly, from one-quarter to one-half a level teaspoonful of salt can be added to each cup of hot water. This will in nearly all cases insure a speedy and satisfactory bowel movement. This, however, is not advised unless absolutely necessary.

It is well to point out that this treatment in its extreme form can hardly be used with complete satisfaction by those who are below average strength. In any case, however, the drinking of a small amount of hot water can be attempted and the exercises illustrated can be used, if one is careful not to make his efforts too severe. The hot-water drinking process as well as the exercise must, however, be adapted to the requirements of each individual, and it may be well in most cases to experiment two or three times before following all of these suggestions in detail.

Where one is lacking in vital strength a beginning can be made by taking only two cups of hot water, using exercises 7, 8 and 9, which can be taken in a reclining position.

One may continue in this way for a week or two, after which a third cup of hot water might be added. In this way one can gradually increase the amount of water consumed and the vigor and the amount of the exercise taken.

Where there is a tendency toward rheumatism, gout, neuritis, neuralgia, or where there are any other symptoms indicating the accumulation of poisons or impurities in the system, it is advisable to use distilled water, though if this cannot be secured ordinary boiled water will be satisfactory. At least be sure to boil your water before using if it is heavily charged with mineral matter, since boiling tends to precipitate lime salts. In other words, hard water is not desirable in such cases.

The hot-water-drinking regimen in itself has a decidedly beneficial effect upon the stomach and intestines. But much better results, especially in the case of constipation, are secured when the special nerve-stimulating exercises recommended are taken in connection with it. By this combination we obtain results that cannot be secured in any other way. In fact, stiffness, soreness and rheumatic "twinges" in various parts of the body are often removed with astounding rapidity through the help of this particular treatment. The cleansing and eliminating functions are stimulated to an extraordinary extent by combining these two blood-purifying forces: hot-water-drinking and the stimulation of the nerve centers.

This regimen is also a splendid means of increasing the weight in cases of defective assimilation. It seems to tone up the entire vital and functional system, in addition to directly influencing the digestive organs. The hot water alone tends to cleanse and empty very thoroughly the stomach and intestines, also to stimulate the secretion of the digestive juices. Those who are below normal weight chiefly because of poor assimilative powers are especially advised to give this method a thorough trial for a period of a few weeks.

Again, if your complexion is sallow, dull, and "muddy," a remarkable improvement will speedily appear as a result of this treatment. In a recent case I observed a surprising change at the end of one week in a complexion that had been sallow and lifeless. The complexion in this instance not only assumed an improved color, but the tissues of the face were also filled out considerably, and when improvement is thus manifested on the surface you can well realize that the internal changes are even more pronounced.

The devitalized condition of the various glands and structures in this part of the body is gradually remedied by the improvement in the circulation that comes with what might be termed a stimulating supply of liquids, and the same good result is accomplished, so far as the general circulation is concerned, in the welfare of the body as a whole. Those suffering from high blood pressure will find this treatment of unusual value, though great care should, of course, be taken to avoid any movements that are in any way exhausting or violent. When the blood is in a thick or viscous condition the use of the hot water adds to its fluidity, and it can then be forced more easily through the capillaries, thus greatly lessening the blood pressure. It is well known that a low blood pressure is conducive to endurance and to general health. And when these exercises especially advised for stimulating the nerve centers and for strengthening and vitalizing the spine are combined with a liberal use of hot water, the blood is forced through all the tissues, with the general effect of thoroughly cleansing all parts, in addition to immediately cleansing the alimentary canal.

It is customary among athletes to use massage, or what is commonly called a "rub down," following their exercise. The purpose of this is to increase the circulation and thereby to carry out of the muscles the fatigue-poisons that have accumulated therein during the exercise. Now if a large amount of hot water is used in connection with movements such as we are illustrating, this purpose will be even more thoroughly accomplished during the exercise itself, as the muscular and other tissues are virtually flushed out owing to the more fluid character of the blood and its more ready and perfect circulation through all parts. One who feels stiff from severe exercise, or finds his tissues sore for other reasons, should be able to overcome this stiffness and gain a sense of refreshment through this method.

Referring to the subject of elimination in the case of fatigue, I might say that some students have ascribed the feeling of fatigue at the end of the day's work to an accumulation of deposits within the walls of the arteries and veins, which deposits are ordinarily carried off during sleep. If this theory is true I can think of no simpler or more satisfactory method of removing this waste matter in the blood-vessels than this system of flushing them. For producing immediate results of any kind there is no other method so far as I know which is so effective as this if one has sufficient strength properly to use it. I have known cases in which a headache has been cured in a few minutes by sprinting or other violent exercise, and cases in which neuralgic toothaches and other pains have yielded to vigorous exercise continued for a prolonged period. I have also known the same relief to be obtained by drinking a liberal quantity of hot water, but in all such instances results would be more quickly and certainly secured through a combination of these stimulating forces.

To repeat for clearness and emphasis, the method outlined consists of the following:

A combination of hot-water-drinking and specially adapted movements for stimulating the nerve centers.

Half a pint to a pint of hot water-as hot as can be drunk-to be taken on beginning the treatment immediately on arising in the morning. An additional quantity of hot water to be taken each five to ten minutes thereafter until from one to two quarts have been consumed.

A large amount of clothing to be worn if profuse perspiration is desired, though where an increase of weight is of advantage and no actual disease exists in the system, no more clothing should be worn than is necessary to maintain warmth.

When a bowel movement is definitely needed, a complete and perfectly satisfactory evacuation is often brought about while taking this treatment. The cleansing process, however, will result in a clearer brain and an improved physical as well as mental capacity, whether or not the bowels act immediately, and one can nearly always depend upon a satisfactory movement later.

When there is suffering from temporary attacks of constipation and immediate relief is desired, add from one-quarter to one-half a level teaspoonful of salt to each cup of hot water. Speedy results can be depended upon in virtually every case. Another method of accomplishing the same thing is to continue the hot-water-drinking even beyond the two quarts suggested, adding no more than a small pinch of salt to each cup, as previously suggested. No harm will come from this excessive water-drinking if one is possessed of a normal amount of vigor.

If one is athletic, jumping one to two hundred times, as when jumping a rope, just previous to moving the bowels is often of value in inducing a natural desire that in nearly all cases brings satisfactory results. Where it is difficult to take the amount of water prescribed, take as much as you conveniently can, gradually increasing the quantity each day.

This hot-water-drinking regimen is not necessarily recommended as a permanent measure to be continued every day for an indefinite period. When you feel that your physical status is satisfactory in every way, you can drop the method for a few days, after which it can be resumed as desired, though it would be of advantage to continue taking the exercises each day, and if even one or two glasses of hot water are taken beneficial results would accrue.

CHAPTER VII: Exercise for Vitality Building

Inactivity is non-existence. It means death. Our bodily powers and organs were given to us for a definite purpose. Failure to use them brings serious penalties. There can be no real health with physical stagnation. To be sure, we may point to some men possessing extraordinary vitality who, apparently, have lived without exercise. But a study of their habits of life will usually bring to light some form of muscular activity, even if it be nothing more than a moderate amount of walking. In some cases, such extraordinary vitality may be possessed that health laws can be broken with apparent impunity, but it will usually be found that a vigorous constitution was developed in early youth from plenty of exercise. However, the failure to observe these important bodily requirements invariably means trouble before reaching the period at which old age begins.

Though the average of human life has been greatly increased through the decline in infant mortality, the death rate among men of middle age has more than doubled in the past thirty years. And even if those of exceptional vitality can neglect their physical requirements without suffering, the man of limited energy, who is trying to build vitality, certainly cannot afford to do so.

We ought to take a reasonable amount of exercise at intervals, regular or otherwise, in order to keep fully alive. It is not a case of exercise for the sake of muscular strength alone, but for the sake of health and life. There are many people who labor under the delusion that they are living without exercise, but existing does not mean living. To live in the full sense of the word means that you are thoroughly alive, and you positively cannot be thoroughly alive unless all the physical processes involved in the various functions of the body are active. Functional activity means pure blood, of superior quality, and when one fails to give the muscular system its proper use, the functions stagnate, the blood is filled with impurities of various sorts, and under such circumstances the body is not really alive. When the body is harboring an excessive number of dead cells and other waste material one cannot say that he is entirely alive. Under such conditions you are literally half dead and half alive. It is well known that the body is dying at all times. Minute cells that constitute the bodily tissues lose their vitality and life, and are taken up by the venous blood and carried to the various organs which take part in the work of elimination. Now these dead cells and minute corpuscles linger in the tissues if one lives an inactive life. Therefore it is literally true that you are half dead if you do not give the muscular system its proper use.

Physically the muscular system is such an important part of the body that failure to keep it in good condition by failure to keep it active seriously affects all other parts. The greater part of the food we eat is consumed by the muscles. Most of the heat produced by the body is generated in the muscles. Therefore to neglect this part of our organism means to disorganize, to a large extent, the workings of all other parts. The appetite, under such conditions, fails and the entire functional system loses tone. In fact, I may say that exercise is the first and most important of all the methods of building functional strength. When the muscles are exercised the vital, organs are energized and the activity of the entire functional system greatly increased-all clearly indicating that in taking physical exercise the internal organs are aroused and stimulated.

Gigantic strength is not especially needed. It is not necessary for one to strive to eclipse the feats of famous strong men. Unusual muscular development is of no great value in this age, but a normal degree of strength is absolutely necessary in the struggle for health and vitality. No one should be satisfied with less than what might be regarded as a normal degree of strength, and this, when once developed, can usually be retained by a moderate amount of exercise each day.

Now it is not necessary to adopt some complicated system of exercise for giving the muscles the required activity. Your exercise can take the form of play. It may preferably be taken out-of-doors. But you must keep definitely in mind that the body was given you for active use, and some regular method must be adopted that will insure the activity required.

The exercises referred to in the chapter on Outdoor Life may first of all be recommended. If you have no bodily defects any one of these outdoor sports will probably give your muscles all the exercise needed, but if you are suffering from defects of any kind and you are desirous of remedying them some special exercises adapted to your individual needs should be taken with religious regularity. If you have a flat or sunken chest, if you are round-shouldered, if there is one shoulder higher than the other, if there is a spinal curvature, or if the muscles of the stomach or abdomen are weak, it will be necessary to give special attention to such parts through systematic movements intended to have a corrective influence. In another part of this volume various exercises have been illustrated that are especially recommended to those who are already in possession of ordinary strength. In this chapter I am illustrating a series of movements that have a similar object in view, but which will be found far easier to perform. The exercises in this chapter are especially adapted to those who are weak or ailing. They are designed, however, for the purpose of stimulating and strengthening the spine, which, as I have previously suggested, is the central source of vitality. The hot-water drinking regimen referred to in the chapter on Cleansing the Alimentary Canal can also be used in connection with these exercises, though naturally if one is weak but a small quantity of water can be taken.

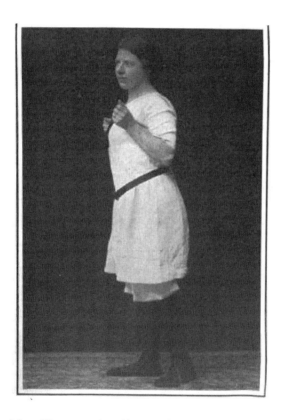

From position illustrated strike straight to the front vigorously.
Return to the first position and then strike downward vigorously.
Return to first position, after which strike upward vigorously as
far as you can reach. Repeat these three exercises, changing from
one to the other until fatigued,

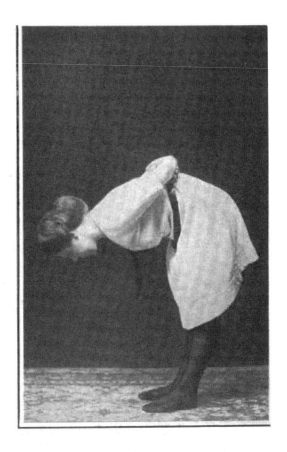

Bend far forward. When you have made the movement to the limit, twist the body far to the right and far to the left, after which return to the erect position. From erect position bend body far to the right. Now while in this position twist the body as far as possible in one direction and then in the other direction. Return to erect position, after which take the same exercise, bending the body far over to the side in the other direction.

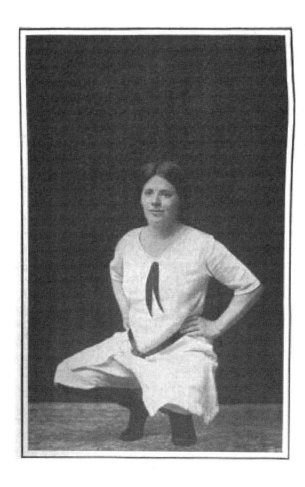

From an erect position, bend the knees until you assume the attitude shown in the above photograph. Return to first position. Repeat until fatigued.

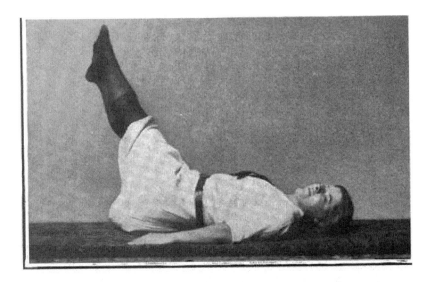

While lying flat on the back with legs fully extended, raise legs to a
perpendicular position, after which sway them far over to the right,
return to the former position and raise the legs again, swaying them far
over to the left. Keep the knees rigid, extend right and left arms far to
the side in order to balance the body while performing this exercise.

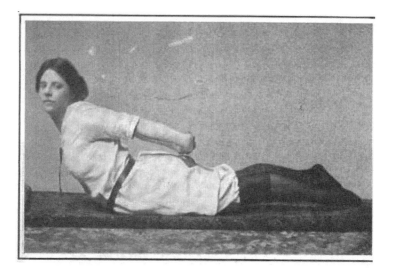

Lie face downward with fingers interlacing behind the back. Raise the body to the position illustrated, or as high as possible. Return to former position and repeat until tired.

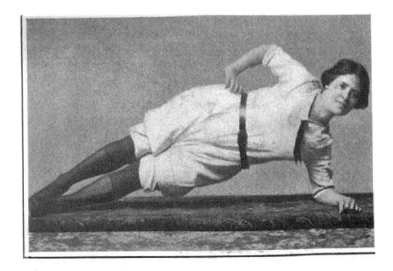

Assume position shown in illustration, now raise the hips as high as you can from the floor. Return to the floor and repeat until fatigued, after which take the same exercise, reversing the position with the right arm on the floor.

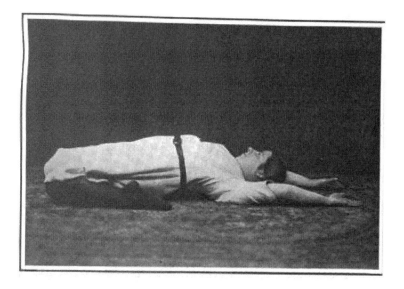

The above photograph illustrates the possibilities in connection with the development of suppleness. After considerable practice almost any one can assume the above attitude from a standing position in what appears to be one continuous movement. While standing drop to the knees, extending the toes back as shown in illustration. One foot should be on each side of the hips. Now bring the body back and stretch the arms far overhead as shown.

CHAPTER VIII: How to Breathe

Volumes have been written upon the value of breathing exercises. Many exaggerated statements have been made as to what can be accomplished through deep breathing. Nevertheless, it must be definitely understood that full, deep breaths, which expand the lungs to their fullest capacity, and are taken at frequent intervals, are of great value.

Almost any vigorous exercise will enforce deep breathing, and there is no question as to the benefit of the involuntary or spontaneous inhalation and exhalation thus induced. Running and wrestling are types of very vigorous athletic exercises that will compel one to breathe deeply and fully, and will insure a full lung development without special breathing exercises. And this is more especially true if much exercise of this character is taken regularly, day after day, all the year round. But where the occupation and surroundings are such that one cannot indulge in such active pastimes, or where the time for such exercises is necessarily limited, frequent voluntary deep-breathing exercises can be highly commended. About the best example of the proper use of the diaphragm and the natural movement of the abdominal and dorsal region in correct breathing is illustrated in a small child. In nearly all cases an active healthy child will breathe properly, and by studying the movement of his abdomen in both standing and reclining positions you will find that as the breath is inhaled the abdominal region will expand. When the breath is exhaled this part of the body will contract or be drawn inward. This demonstrates very conclusively that the movement or expansion of the body in natural breathing is abdominal, and that the bony framework of the chest should not be involved except when taking full deep breaths, or when breathing hard from the effects of very vigorous exercise.

It is not at all necessary to go through a complicated system in order to learn proper methods of breathing, since this is comparatively simple if you are willing to make persistent efforts day after day until you are fittingly rewarded. If you simply acquire the habit of drawing in a deep full breath, at frequent intervals during the day, expanding first in the abdominal region, you will soon be able to breathe properly. A correct position of the body is very important, for if you have the proper erect posture, and have no constricting clothing about the waist and abdominal region, you will almost instinctively be inclined to breathe diaphragmatically, or abdominally, as we call it. Furthermore, when going out in the open air you will find as a result of this practice that you are unconsciously expanding in the proper manner as suggested. In fact, you will be more inclined to breathe freely and deeply at all times if a proper position is maintained. It is hardly necessary to mention the necessity for breathing pure air, and especially when taking deep-breathing exercises, if you wish the very greatest results. Take these deep breaths when in the open air, or else before an open window. It is a good plan, for instance, when rising in the morning to stand before an open window and inhale perhaps a dozen full, complete breaths. This will help greatly to brush the cobwebs from your brain and brighten you up for the day's duties and responsibilities.

All of these suggestions apply with equal force to both sexes. Because of the fashions of dress usually in vogue the breathing of women is much more restricted than that of men. Furthermore, they are generally less inclined to athletic pursuits involving exercise which compels deep breathing.

The method of breathing recommended for women is absolutely identical with that suggested for men. It is a curious fact that until recent years the world generally, the medical profession included, held the opinion that there is a fundamental difference between men and women in breathing. Observation of the natural breathing of boys and girls would soon prove the absurdity of this opinion. Owing to the universal use of the corset, thoracic breathing, or chest breathing, the result of the artificial constriction of the body at and below the waist line, appeared to be the natural method of breathing for women, whereas diaphragmatic breathing was recognized as proper and natural for men. Only in recent years have medical authorities recognized that this difference was really due only to artificial methods of dress and that natural breathing in women and men is absolutely the same. Recent

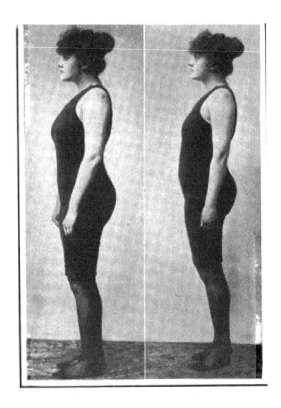

The figure to the left shows the position with the abdomen drawn in when the breath is exhaled. The figure to the right shows the position when the abdomen is expanded by a full breath. In full diaphragmatic breathing, the movement should be confined to the abdominal region though deep breathing exercises expanding the chest to the fullest extent can be practiced with benefit.

fashions have permitted the enlargement of the waist line in women, but unfortunately there is still too much constriction of this important part of the body. When the world becomes more truly civilized and our methods of dress are based upon common sense and an intelligent understanding of the physical requirements of the body, we may hope that the dress of women will be such as to permit entire freedom in the matter of breathing, and the easy expansion of the body at the waist line. Some day women will learn the value of suspending skirts, stockings, etc., from the shoulders instead of relying upon the restriction at the waist as a means of support.

If you wish to ascertain more exactly whether or not your breathing is entirely satisfactory, stand up, take a deep breath, and observe not only the expansion in the region of the stomach and abdomen but also at the sides and in the back. If you place the palms of your hands upon the lower ribs in the back, just above the waist line, you should feel the expansion of the body in this part pressing upward through the action of the diaphragm as a deep breath is inhaled. Also by pressing the hands upon the lower ribs at the sides, just above the waist line, you will feel the lateral expansion in this region at the same time that the expansion is noted in the front of the body. You will therefore realize that there should be an expansion of the lower ribs at the back and at the sides along with the expansion in the region of the stomach and abdomen. Of course, when a very full breath is taken there will also be an expansion of the chest following the filling up of the lower part of the lungs.

CHAPTER IX: Outdoor Life

Civilized man is an indoor animal. We no longer live in tree-tops nor even in caves, but in houses, and a great many of us spend the larger part of every year in close, ill-ventilated, overheated rooms. From a health viewpoint the cave-dweller would no doubt have the advantage over the average American who follows a sedentary occupation. The steam-heated apartments of our great cities are thoroughly aired only on rare intervals, and consequently those who reside therein often dry up in mind, soul and body along with the furniture.

In order to live in every sense of the word we must become a part of the great outdoors. Outdoor life adds to one's vitality and vigor. It increases one's energies and enthusiasms. You cannot be ambitious or vivacious, you cannot really amount to anything in life, if you are confined to an overheated flat.

If there is any hobby that is worth while it is one that takes us out-of-doors. What the attractive features of your hobby may be, is not of very great importance provided this object is secured. You must be lured away from your stuffy living rooms and encouraged to breathe the fresh, pure air of the open.

There are out-of-door exercises of all sorts which are of great value, but even a seat in a motor car wherein your exercise is confined principally to increased respiration through the pleasure that comes with fast riding, is at least of some value. The health of the nation, as a whole, has been greatly improved by the automobile through its encouragement of the outdoor life. But if you can join with your outdoor life some active exercise which will use all the muscles of the body the benefits will be much greater.

There are various open-air pastimes that can be made unusually vigorous, and so can be highly recommended if one is possessed of ordinary strength. Football is perhaps one of the most strenuous of outdoor games, and is to be especially advised where one has the vitality and endurance which fits him for an exercise of this character.

Golf is an example of a milder outdoor pastime that is particularly suited to middle-aged and elderly persons, although young men and women are benefited by it, too. It affords excellent exercise in walking, and the swinging of the golf clubs affords more exercise for the chest, arms and back than is usually supposed. One who is not accustomed to the game will usually find the muscles of the arms, shoulders and chest sore or at least stiff from the unusual exercise when first attempting to play this game.

Tennis furnishes a vigorous exercise that is especially commendable for adding to one's vitality. It is a good endurance builder. Tennis can be made as fast and energetic, or as leisurely and moderate as one wishes, depending entirely upon the skill, strength and ability of the player. Tennis is a safe and sane pastime that is growing in popularity, and can be universally recommended for both sexes and all ages.

Rowing, running, cross-country work, track athletics, lacrosse, handball, hockey and polo are all splendid and vigorous games, well calculated to develop the best type of physical stamina. For those possessing the requisite strength they can all be highly recommended, though as a rule it is best not to specialize in any one of them but to secure as much variety as possible. Specializing in athletics may win championships and may stimulate interest in sports, but for the average man or woman specialization is not desirable. Even if you are only a "dub" instead of a champion in each of these games, it is better to play them all, since you will thereby secure a well-rounded physical development, and also obtain the maximum of "fun."

For those who are less rugged but who on that very account are all the more in need of open-air exercise there is a great variety of other less strenuous pastimes. Cycling and horseback riding can be particularly recommended as enjoyable forms of outing in combination with a certain amount of exercise. Skating is an ideal pastime for the colder weather as it requires no special strength and adds to the vigor of the heart, lungs and other vital organs; besides this, the brisk, cold air of the winter months is a tonic of great value. Snowshoeing, yachting, rope-skipping, canoeing, archery, croquet, coasting and various similar pastimes are all to be commended.

Swimming is of great value, both as a means of physical development and as a health builder, but if your vitality is limited do not stay in the water too long. Swimming may be made mild or very strenuous. If you swim with the skill of an expert, only a very moderate exertion is required, though some of the new racing strokes tax the strength and endurance of the strongest athlete. Swimming combines the pleasures of bathing and exercise, and under proper conditions is invaluable. Those who are "fleshy" can stay in the water a long time, but if you are "thin" take care lest you lose weight by too much bathing. The slender man or woman may take a daily swim for its tonic effect. It may even cause one to gain in weight if the exercise is not prolonged, but persons of this type usually lose weight in the course of a season of too much bathing.

There is one point of special importance in connection with our exercise and that is to cultivate the play spirit. You will never fully enjoy your sports and you will never obtain all possible benefit from them until you lose your dignity and learn how to play. Try to be glad that you are alive and able to play these games. One great drawback to American sports is the tendency to take them too seriously. There is too much of strained effort involved in the desire to win the game at any price. Keep yourself in a state of mind where you "see the fun." Though "playing to win" may be commended, the real purpose of any game is the fun and benefit that is secured therefrom whether you win or lose. There have been cases when members of a boat crew or a football team have actually cried over a lost game. Imagine the nerve strain involved in taking athletics so seriously! It is splendid to win, but it should also be pleasurable to lose to a worthy antagonist. Do not take your games too seriously, but make them a laughing matter. Only by assuming this attitude can you get the greatest possible benefits that can be derived from games. The nature of your exercise does not matter so long as there is that increased activity of the heart, lungs and other organs which tends to improve the circulation throughout the entire body. The exercise must insure deep breathing, and if a certain amount of perspiration is induced it will be advantageous. First of all get out-of-doors; find some exercise that appeals, some alluring attraction which will take you away from the confinement of your home. Live as much as you can in the open. If possible, try sleeping out-of-doors. Men and women of today may be aptly compared to sensitive plants. We are the devitalized product of the universal custom of coddling, and the less we live within four walls, and the more we breathe the free outdoor air, the stronger, healthier and more capable we become.

There is one outdoor exercise that we can all take without expense, and it is by far the best when everything is considered. At least this statement is true so far as the building of vitality and endurance is concerned. I refer to walking. This is an exercise that can be made decidedly vigorous if desired. And no matter what health-building regimen you may follow, a certain amount of walking is essential to maintaining the highest degree of physical vigor.

Walking is a tonic of very great value to every one of the organic functions. It stimulates the activities of the purifying organs to an unusual degree. It is a remedy of great efficacy in overcoming constipation. It can be highly recommended for strengthening the heart, for stimulating the liver and kidneys, and it will tone up the physical organism throughout. Furthermore, this exercise is of unusual value as a mental stimulant. It clears the "cobwebs" from the brain. If you are bothered with vexing problems put them aside until you can take a long walk. With the improved quality of the blood and the more active circulation of this functional tonic, your mental efficiency will be greatly increased. You will think more quickly; your conclusions will be clearer, more definite and more dependable. I know a successful novelist who depends very largely upon his long walks for working out the themes and plots of his stories. I have frequently followed the same plan in connection with my own work. I know of other writers who depend upon this method of gaining inspiration. I have been told that chopping wood is mentally stimulating, and also that horseback riding and cycling are sometimes helpful in this direction, but walking is without doubt the most effective mental stimulant to be found out-of-doors. It accelerates the circulation, and seems to arouse the vital forces of the body, but does not require such an expenditure of energy as to prevent the brain from being exceptionally active.

Now to secure the real benefits that come from walking there should be no laziness about it. Do not walk as though you were on a fashion parade. The Sunday afternoon stroll on the city streets may be very alluring, but you cannot under such circumstances secure the real benefits that may be found in walking. If possible go out on the country roads or walk across the fields. Put a certain amount of energy into your every step. Walk briskly and as though you enjoyed it, and you will discover that you do enjoy it. Even if your first few steps require an unusual effort on your part, "step lively" just the same, and you will shortly find that you feel lively, too. A walk of this sort into which you put real energy in every step is a tonic of amazing value. It will stir up your entire organism. It will insure an active functioning, and make you feel and be thoroughly alive. If you have the added advantage that comes from pure country air you are to be envied. But even without these superior advantages, even if your route is confined to city streets, some benefit will still result from taking the walk tonic.

While walking give special attention to my suggestions concerning breathing. Breathe deeply and fully at frequent intervals. Expand the body in the abdominal region. If you like, you can carry your breathing still farther and allow this expansion to extend to the chest walls, though as a rule, this is not necessary. No doubt one of the most valuable suggestions for strength and vitality building while walking is to take at frequent periods several movements which are referred to in the chapter on Thyroid Stimulation, namely, the chin-in-downward-and-backward motion while holding a full breath with abdomen fully expanded. In fact this idea, if carried out until the muscles of the back of the neck are fatigued at the completion of the walk, will energize you mentally and physically. A suggestion that I have often offered in various articles upon this subject is to practice what I may term harmonious or rhythmic breathing, which I regard as of exceptional value. By this I mean taking the same amount of time to draw in the breath as you do to exhale it, keeping time with a certain number of steps. For instance, while taking eight steps, draw in a breath and exhale during the next eight steps. You may make this six, eight, ten or twelve steps if you like. If you have some piece of music in mind that carries with it a rhythm that accommodates itself to your steps while walking, and if each inhalation and exhalation takes up an even number of steps, you will find that you are swinging along with a sense of harmony and pleasure that will make distances pass away and cause you to be unconscious of the length of your walk. This rhythmic or harmonious breathing is an excellent means of cultivating the deep-breathing habit.

Another exercise is of material value in connection with the practice of deep breathing while walking, serving especially to stimulate the digestive and other internal organs. This consists in holding a fairly full breath for a series of four, six or eight steps, and at the same time expanding the body still further in the region of the stomach. This is accomplished largely through the action of the diaphragm and the muscles across the front of the body in the region of the stomach. This should be executed with a sort of pumping motion, that is to say by a series of alternate contractions and relaxations rapidly following each other. Expand the region of the stomach by this muscular effort for an instant, relax, repeat, and continue in that way several times during the course of the six or eight steps during which you hold the breath. Then exhale freely and after one or two breaths repeat. This has the effect of massaging, as it were, the internal organs, and is of material value in bringing about improved functioning, as well as strengthening these parts.

If you can find an opportunity to go camping there is no better way in which to spend a vacation. Everyone knows that a term of two or three weeks in the woods or by the side of a lake, living out-of-doors to some extent after the manner of primitive man, and getting a certain amount of pleasurable exercise with the continuous fresh air, will work wonders.

But if camping for a short period is beneficial, then a part of each day in the open air during the summer is well worth while; therefore try to "camp out" for two or three hours each evening. If you are through work at five o'clock, for instance, enjoy a picnic dinner in the open, instead of a regular supper in the dining-room of your home. It is daylight until almost eight o'clock during most of the summer, and this plan would yield two or three hours of open-air life. Or take advantage of part of this time, before supper, to go rowing, or swimming, to play some game, such as tennis, or to do anything else that will occupy you pleasantly for an hour or two in the open air. At least you can always take a good walk. If you go to bed at a reasonable hour you can probably rise early enough to permit a walk of one or two hours, or some other open-air activity, before going to work. If your work is in an office where you will be confined all day this advice is especially important. When your office hours begin at eight or nine o'clock in the morning you should imbibe as much fresh air as possible before work, if only by walking part or all the way to your place of business. Be in the open air as much as you can. Many people think they are too busy for this. They make the plea of lack of time, but when illness appears they have plenty of time to stay in bed. The open-air man or woman "side-steps" sickness. Since superabundant vitality can be obtained through open-air life, spend as much time as you can out-of-doors. Cultivate the outdoor habit. It will increase your efficiency so that you will do better work in less time.

CHAPTER X: Strengthening the Stomach

One of the first requirements in vitality building is strengthening the stomach. Within the stomach we find the beginning of all vital blood-making processes. Here is where the food first passes through the changes essential to create the life-building fluid called the blood. We therefore cannot exaggerate the importance of strength to this important organ. When referring to a strong stomach, I do not mean strength in the abdominal muscles lying immediately in front of the stomach; I mean strength of the muscles within the walls of the stomach itself, which, to a large extent, actually constitute the stomach. These layers of muscular fibers which assist in carrying on important parts of the digestive processes must be strong if digestion is to be satisfactory in every way.

Now the work of strengthening the stomach does not, by any means, consist wholly of exercise. The stomach in order to be strengthened must have a due amount of intelligent consideration at all times. For instance, you cannot make a garbage can of your stomach and expect to increase the strength of the organ. It is really necessary, if you are seriously desirous of securing the best results in vitality building, to learn at least the fundamental facts relating to rational dietetics; and, after acquiring this knowledge, to apply it to your individual use throughout every day of your life. The suggestions that I have offered in the chapter on Cleansing and Stimulating the Alimentary Canal are truly of extreme importance in these strengthening processes. In fact in every instance this plan will increase the assimilative strength, and will enable you to create a better quality of blood; and this result in turn naturally aids in strengthening the stomach itself as well as all other parts of the body. Furthermore, this is a method for cleansing directly not only the organ itself but the various glands which furnish the digestive juices. Therefore, if difficulties are frequently presented in connection with the functions of this organ, special attention should be given to the elemental cleansing and strengthening processes as outlined in the chapter referred to.

There are various special exercises which will have a certain influence upon the stomach because of their mechanical stimulation of this organ. All bending and twisting movements of the trunk of the body will naturally stimulate the action of the stomach because of their direct mechanical effect. All movements of this sort are naturally valuable under the circumstances, though for a short time after a meal any exercise that is so severe as to interfere with digestion should be avoided. Such interference results when the muscles are used to such an extent that they require greatly increased quantities of blood at a time when a plentiful supply is needed by the stomach to carry on the work of digestion. All my readers no doubt already understand the necessity for giving the digestive organs every opportunity to carry on their processes for at least one hour after a hearty meal. Bending and body-twisting movements are valuable one hour or more after a meal for strengthening the stomach, but they interfere with digestion if taken immediately thereafter. For increasing the vigor of this most important organ I would especially recommend the method already referred to for cleansing the alimentary canal and also the exercises which are given in connection therewith in the same chapter. If one is not in possession of a fair amount of strength I would suggest merely the exercises illustrated in Chapter VII to be taken in conjunction with the morning hot-water-drinking regimen.

It should be remembered, however, that for the strengthening of the stomach one must really depend most of all upon a proper diet and the care of the stomach generally, rather than upon any system of exercises intended to invigorate this organ.

To build up a strong stomach a daily plan of life must be followed which requires of the entire body a normal amount of activity, thus demanding and using a fairly liberal supply of nourishment. An active life is always favorable to good digestion, and especially so if it is an out-of-door life for at least a large part of each day, for then an appetite is created demanding of the stomach that healthy activity essential to strength building; in other words, an active and normal life generally is essential to the maintenance of a strong and healthy stomach. The body must be regarded not as an aggregation of parts, but as one complete unit, and anything that affects all parts affects each separate part. It is quite true that when the stomach is weakened from any cause, it is not wise to overtax it by the ingestion of foods that are difficult to digest. But at the same time a policy of using predigested foods, or others that are suited only to a weak stomach, is not likely to develop a vigorous digestion. It is essential that one should use a proper supply of natural and wholesome foods properly prepared. If this is done and the general rules of rational dietetics are observed, there is no reason why any one should not enjoy the possession of a strong stomach and a vigorous digestion. I cannot, however, place too much emphasis upon the value of outdoor life and general activity and the constitutional benefits that go with them for improving the stomach as well as all other parts of the body.

CHAPTER XI: Preserving the Teeth

Health to a large extent depends upon the teeth. Food can not be properly masticated without sound molars. The modern tendency of teeth to decay early in life clearly proves that something is wrong with our dietetic or chewing habits. Like any other part of the body, the teeth must be exercised in order to be properly preserved. Our foods are so frequently macerated to a fine consistency and they are so often cooked to a mush before they are eaten, that the teeth have little to do. They decay and become soft or brittle because of lack of use.

It is necessary to give the teeth a reasonable amount of regular use. Cultivate the habit of eating zwieback, hard crackers or other hard food substances that require real vigorous chewing. If this is difficult, then make a habit of exercising the teeth in some way. The idea suggested in the illustrations accompanying this chapter will be found of value, though any method can be recommended that serves the same purpose. Do not, however, depend upon the chewing of gum for hours each day as a means of exercising the teeth. Chewing a hard gum for a few minutes after a meal might be of advantage, but continual gum-chewing wastes and weakens the digestive elements of the saliva. In other words, if you sit down to a meal after chewing gum for two or three hours, the saliva that you mix with your food will not have the normal digestive elements. One might say that the "strength" of the saliva has been lost while chewing gum.

If your teeth are decayed the offending members should be removed or the cavities filled. It is always wise to retain every tooth you can until extraction is practically compulsory. Decayed teeth should be filled promptly. As long as a tooth can be filled it should not be extracted. A good dentist should be consulted at frequent intervals.

If tartar has collected on the teeth, it should be removed by a competent dentist. One good method of keeping the teeth free from tartar is to rub the gums and teeth daily with table salt containing considerable grit. Dampen the finger, place a quantity of table salt thereon and then rub the teeth where they meet the gums. Make the process sufficiently vigorous to rub off any tartar that may have accumulated. The mouth should be rinsed with moderately warm water immediately after this process to remove the salt. Any good tooth wash that is sold in the form of paste can be used instead of salt for this same purpose. This rubbing process is of more value to strengthen the gums and to cleanse the teeth than brushing the teeth with an ordinary tooth brush.

Tooth brushes, however, are valuable and should be used morning and evening. In caring for the teeth the following plan is suggested:

Soon after rising rinse the mouth out thoroughly with a mild antiseptic tooth wash; soap, or salt and water, is fairly good if nothing better can be obtained. Plain water will also serve the purpose. Lemon juice to which considerable water has been added, also makes a good mouth wash. Orange juice can also be recommended.

It may be said that most of the standard tooth powders and tooth pastes on the market at the present time are fairly reliable and satisfactory, particularly those of which the formula is printed on the wrapper. When brushing the teeth, avoid using a brush with the bristles too hard. A medium- or even a soft-bristle brush is preferable. The lateral action of the tooth brush, commonly used, is of limited value. One should use a vertical or up-and-down movement, so that the bristles will reach the crevices between the teeth. It is the spaces between the teeth that particularly need cleaning and the brush should be used in such a way as to reach these. It is here that decay usually begins.

After having brushed the teeth then rub them in the manner previously described. Spend two or three or even four or five minutes at this rubbing process. If the teeth are free from tartar do not use the salt more than once or twice weekly, though any good tooth paste could be used daily to advantage, not for brushing the teeth, mind you, but for rubbing the gums and teeth.

For removing accumulated food substances from between the teeth silk or linen floss can be recommended. Holding the thread between the fingers of each hand force it down between two teeth and bring it back

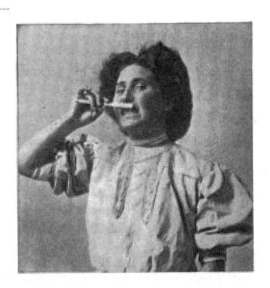

Illustrating how the toothbrush should be used. Brush the upper teeth downward from the gums and the lower teeth upward from the gums. When the teeth are brushed in this manner the bristles enter the crevices and cleanse the teeth more thoroughly.

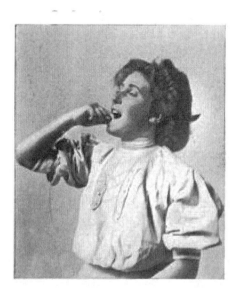

Illustrating a splendid method of massaging the gums with the thumb and first finger. Press the upper gums downward against the teeth and the lower gums upward against the teeth. This massage process is especially advised when using an antiseptic mouth wash.

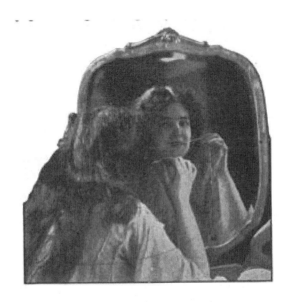

Illustrating the use of silk floss for removing the debris from between the teeth. Force the floss between each of the teeth and pull it forward and backward until all foreign matter has been removed from between the teeth.

and forth. If you have no regular dental floss, use any white silk thread for the purpose. It does not do one much good to brush the teeth if he does not remove decaying and acid-forming matter from between the teeth. The use of dental floss is fully as important as the use of a tooth brush. Where Rigg's disease, or pyorrhea, is present, an antiseptic can be used to advantage two or three times daily after rubbing or washing the teeth. Massage of the gums may prove helpful, if gently applied, though in a serious case of pyorrhea a fasting and general blood-purifying regimen is advisable.

The condition of the teeth is influenced to a large extent by the state of the stomach. Where the digestion is perfect, the breath free from all foul odors, the teeth are less liable to decay and tartar rarely accumulates. Where there is any stomach disorder, however, very great care must be taken to avoid a number of unpleasant symptoms associated with the gradual deterioration of the teeth. If the various suggestions I have made in this volume for maintaining superior health are followed with a reasonable amount of care, and the tooth brush is used regularly, in addition to proper attention being given to thorough mastication, the teeth should be retained as long as there is use for them. Remember, however, the very important suggestion made in another chapter in reference to the value of fruit acid in cleansing the mouth and teeth. If you will rinse the mouth out at frequent intervals with the juice of an orange or eat part or all of an orange, you will be surprised at the cleansing influence of this acid fruit. Almost any acid fruit will be of value, but the orange is perhaps the best for this purpose. The free use of water to insure alimentary cleanliness together with the acid fruit habit will form a very superior insurance for our teeth.

Finally, and of not least importance, the character of the diet has a great influence on the teeth. You cannot keep the teeth sound and strong if the foods you eat do not contain the material out of which teeth are built. If the food elements that build teeth and bone are lacking, you cannot expect the teeth to last long. A great hue and cry has been raised about the poor teeth of the school children of to-day, and an effort is being made to teach the children to brush their teeth. Of course this is good as far as it goes, but it does not go far when the children are fed

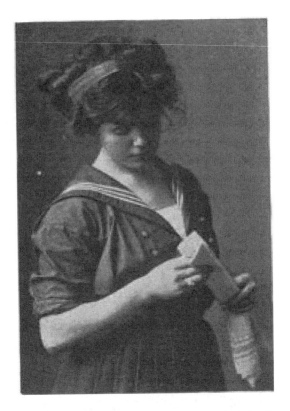

Showing how a small towel can be folded until it is the width of the mouth. This towel can then be used with splendid effect for exercising the teeth.

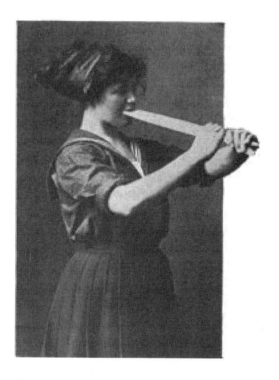

Illustrating the use of the folded towel. After having folded the towel, firmly grip the teeth upon one end of the towel very tightly. While gripping the towel tightly in this manner you can pull upward and downward, to left and right. If these teeth exercises are taken with a certain amount of regularity, they should be of unusual benefit.

upon a diet that is defective. When you find the child of a poor family given a diet of little more than white bread and coffee you can absolutely depend upon it that his teeth are crumbling and decaying. No other result is possible, no matter if the greatest of care is used to keep the teeth well brushed and clean.

Therefore, my remarks in another chapter upon the influence of refined foods will apply particularly in the case of the teeth. A satisfactory supply of lime in the diet is especially necessary for building teeth and bone. Whole-wheat bread will supply the material for building sound teeth, while oatmeal and other whole grain foods are almost equally satisfactory for this purpose.

Some women lose their teeth rapidly as a result of pregnancy, because the diet upon which they live is really a starvation diet so far as these important elements are concerned. Eggs are rich in lime and elements required for building strong teeth, while vegetables and fruits in their natural state are valuable in this way. Good milk is of value for its supply of lime and other organic minerals in the case of young children. Furthermore, all natural foods that provide good exercise for the teeth through the necessity for mastication are valuable on this account for strengthening the teeth, as I have already said.

Dentistry is one of our most useful professions. But there would be need for few dentists if the suggestions given in this chapter were closely followed by men, women and children the whole country over. One may have strong teeth in practically every instance, as a result of proper care and suitable diet, just as he may have strong muscles, strong organs and strong nerves.

CHAPTER XII: How to Eat

Civilization has brought with it a train of evils unknown in the natural life. There is no need, for instance, to tell a wild animal what to eat; his life is planned for him in advance. His food is supplied by Nature and not super-abundantly, so he is compelled to eat it in a manner to secure the greatest amount of vital vigor therefrom. Hunger controls his eating, and therefore he always enjoys his food. If we were to eliminate many of the mechanical processes involved in the preparation of our foods, there would be little or no necessity for instruction in eating, for, if we ate our food in a natural state, we would be compelled to masticate it, and this is the fundamental requirement of healthy digestion.

Just here let me point out the importance of appetite. A food cannot possibly be of benefit unless it is thoroughly enjoyed. It must taste good. The more delicious a food tastes the more quickly and advantageously it will digest. The idea is frequently advanced that dieting must necessarily be unpleasant, for many think that a "diet" must consist of food that cannot possibly be eaten with enjoyment. This is a great mistake. Diet of this character would indeed bring about harmful results in nearly every instance. The diet which will be of the most value is that which you can enjoy, confining your selection, of course, to wholesome articles of food. I cannot emphasize too strongly the extreme necessity for the enjoyment of your meals. Do not under any circumstance ignore the demands of your taste in selecting your diet.

Your food must be thoroughly masticated as well as thoroughly enjoyed. This chewing should continue until the food becomes a liquid and actually passes down your throat involuntarily. Food should never be swallowed hastily. Swallowing should be an unconscious process associated with enjoyment; with a view to prolonging the pleasure of eating, each mouthful should be retained in the mouth until it is swallowed before you realize it. Thorough mastication is absolutely necessary to the attainment of the very important requirements connected with the complete enjoyment of foods.

Now note the effect of prolonged enjoyment of food upon the digestive processes. When one is masticating an appetizing meal the digestive system is being prepared for the reception of this meal. The various glands of the stomach that perform such important work in digestion begin to pour their juices into the stomach; consequently when the food reaches this organ everything is ready for its reception. To begin with, as a result of thorough mastication and the action of the saliva, the food is already partly digested, and the stomach is ready to continue the process. The work is easy and satisfactory under such circumstances, and digestion continues unconsciously. You do not realize that you have a stomach. How often one hears a healthy man say that he has no conscious knowledge of the possession of such an organ! In other words, he has never had a pain or other unpleasant symptom located in its region. It is said on the other hand that the dyspeptic is so continuously and unpleasantly aware of the existence of this organ that he often thinks he is "all stomach."

Remember also the importance of a suitable mental attitude at meal-time. Your mind should be occupied almost entirely with the pleasure of the meal itself. You should not be seriously diverted in any way. If for instance you are reading a newspaper or carrying on an engrossing conversation you are directly interfering with the digestive processes; for, as I have already said, a thorough enjoyment of the food is necessary to arouse to their greatest activity the glands which furnish the digestive juices. Therefore, when meal-time comes around, devote yourself to the one single purpose of getting as much enjoyment as possible out of your food.

If you are desirous of catching a train, do not make the mistake of bolting a meal. Eat when you arrive at your destination, or eat on the train, when you can have the leisure to enjoy your food. Remember that, with eating as with work, it is not how much but how well. If your time is limited it is better to eat only a small amount, and eat it properly, than to attempt to eat a large meal hurriedly.

Especially do not eat when you are angry or worried; do not allow anything to distract you at meal-time. If anything comes up that seriously mars your ability to enjoy your food it is far better to delay your meal or wait until the next meal, or until you can eat in accordance with these requirements.

There can be no objection to light conversation, which requires no special amount of mental energy or concentration; in other words, any deviation can be recommended which does not seriously interfere with the enjoyment of your meal. Music, for instance, if it is of a gentle, soothing character, or entertainment of any kind that is relaxing, is a helpful form of recreation. The "cabaret," if not carried to an extreme, is therefore a natural, well-founded institution. Congenial company is also naturally advantageous in helping one to enjoy his meals.

There has been much controversy as to whether or not one should drink during a meal. I have at all times condemned the usual habit of drinking at meal-time for the purpose of washing down food that is eaten hastily. For instance, it is not at all unusual with many people to take three or four mouthfuls of food, hastily swallow them, and then find a certain amount of liquid essential to avoid choking. I cannot too emphatically condemn a habit of this sort. I do, however, recommend the use of liquids during a meal when they are necessary to satisfy thirst. Furthermore, it is of considerable importance to take some liquid during a meal if one is not in the habit of drinking freely of water between meals, since a certain amount of liquid is necessary to carry on the digestive process. When there is any digestive difficulty or when there is merely a weak digestion, hot water can be used to great advantage fifteen minutes or a half-hour before the meal. Taking hot water in this manner cleanses the stomach and adds materially to the digestive capacity by stimulating the glands of the stomach. The quantity of water taken in this way may range from half a pint to a quart, depending upon one's physical condition. The amount of liquid taken during a meal must also be regulated by one's needs. For instance, if you are poorly nourished and apparently need more weight properly to round out your body, then an additional amount of liquid will often be of advantage, provided you do not take so much as actually to interfere with digestion. Where increased bodily tissue is needed, therefore, in virtually every instance the free use of water during the meal will be of decided value; though one should always keep in mind the necessity of drinking these liquids warm or even hot if taking any quantity.

The use of a large amount of cold water at meal-time is likely to be detrimental. There is a wide-spread custom of drinking ice-water during the meal. This is one of the most pernicious of all dietetic errors, since chilling of the stomach invariably retards digestion and favors dyspepsia. Even water that is very cold, though not iced, is not desirable, unless used in very small amounts. Also the use of ice-water or extremely cold water between meals is inadvisable, since because of its low temperature one cannot comfortably drink enough of it to satisfy completely his bodily requirements. Water that is only moderately cold or cool can be used liberally, and is always to be preferred in the case of overheating through violent exercise. It is usually advisable to drink water at the temperature that is most pleasant to you, though large quantities of cold water should always be avoided. And, as I have said, at meal-time, especially, if much water or other liquids are used they should be either warm or hot.

Without question, the greatest of all dietetic errors is to eat without appetite. It is nothing less than a crime against the stomach, and yet this practice is one of the most common of all those which contribute to the prevalence of dyspepsia in civilized communities. No animal, the human race excepted, would attempt to eat without the relish that absolutely depends upon the possession of a keen appetite. Many thousands of people attempt to eat their meals regularly without regard to the demands of hunger merely because it is "meal-time." Eating in such cases has only the excuse of habit, although frequently it is regarded as a duty. Eating should never be regarded as a duty, nor should it be allowed to become a habit, for when not pleasurable it is not beneficial.

One will often, hear the remark that one must "eat to keep up his strength." While this advice is fundamentally sound in a large sense under normal conditions and when a true appetite is present, yet there never was a greater delusion when it is applied to forced eating when the appetite is lacking. Eating under such conditions does not keep up one's strength, but on the contrary actually impairs it by burdening the digestive system with food that cannot be properly assimilated. It is not what you eat but what you assimilate that keeps you strong, and digestion depends upon appetite and the enjoyment associated therewith. The question of enjoyment is really a question of appetite, and if you are not hungry and cannot relish the food keenly when meal-time comes it is certainly best to wait until the next meal or until you are hungry. Every wild animal has sense enough to follow its natural inclination in this respect, but thousands of human beings go to the table because it is dinner-time, and force themselves to eat food that they do not desire simply because of the stupid delusion that continual and frequent eating is necessary for strength.

The discussion of appetite brings up the question of the number of meals that is proper for each day. The prevailing system of three meals per day is a custom surviving from a time in which early rising and hard physical labor throughout a long day was the rule, especially in connection with out-of-door work. This does not mean, however, that three meals is always the best plan for civilized life in sedentary occupations. There are some wild races that eat only two meals per day, and there have been instances of hunters and even whole populations following the one-meal-per-day plan. Naturally at the present time the occupation and the requirements of the individual would have much to do with the question. If one does hard work, has an appetite for three meals per day, and seems to thrive on that plan, it is the preferable one. If, however, you are a sedentary worker, and especially if you do not have an appetite for three meals per day and cannot thoroughly enjoy them, the two-meal-per-day plan would be much better. The two-meal-per-day plan has often proven beneficial even when associated with the strenuous physical training required for athletic competition in racing, wrestling, boxing, Marathon running and other vigorous sports. It is entirely a question of appetite. If you have no appetite for breakfast then follow the two-meal-per-day plan. I will say, however, that in many cases one can enjoy and profit by a breakfast of fruit.

The question of how to eat is closely related to the question of how many meals one should take. Overeating is a very prevalent failing. There is no question that large numbers eat themselves, as it were, into a condition of stupor. Their energies are required for the disposal of the excessive quantity of food ingested, and they have no energy left for mental work or for physical activity. They are, so to speak, "food drunk." I am personally satisfied that the best cure for overeating is food in less frequent meals and the practice of masticating the food thoroughly in the manner that I have suggested. In a case of this kind the two-meal-per-day plan is also to be recommended. Actual experience shows that those inclined to overeat do not eat any more at one meal when eating two meals than when eating three meals-they may possibly eat less, because of the more normal condition of the stomach. Another good plan to pursue is the use of uncooked foods, or at least the adoption of a diet consisting in part of uncooked foods. It is entirely possible to eat too little of nourishing food, just as it is to eat too much. But one who lives a natural and active life, especially if out-of-doors a fair part of the time, is not likely to lack a good appetite nor to eat less than the required amount. Good general health always brings with it a normal appetite.

Overeating, however, is no doubt in many cases due very largely to the inadequate character of the foods consumed. I am satisfied that if all our foods were eaten in their natural condition and if they perfectly supplied the needs of the body there would be no tendency toward overeating. The great trouble is that conventional methods of food preparation have such a destructive effect upon the nutritive value of the foods in common use that a healthy body often craves large quantities of diverse foods in order to get a sufficiency of certain elements which are lacking. The use of white bread is a case in point, for, as stated in another chapter, the best part of the wheat has been eliminated in the process of milling. Furthermore, to a large extent the mineral salts are removed from our vegetables in the process of boiling; that is to say, when the water in which they were boiled is thrown away. The polishing of rice, the use of white flour in manufacturing macaroni, the refining of our sugar, and many other processes, are directly responsible for the almost universal habit of overeating.

Certain elements are taken out of the food, the body craves these elements, and in trying to secure adequate nourishment, one eats an excessive amount of the refined defective foods.

CHAPTER XIII: What to Eat

The suggestions offered in the previous chapter concerning the necessity for the enjoyment of food, give one a fairly clear idea as to what he should eat. In other words, he should select those foods that he thoroughly enjoys, keeping in mind the necessity of using only those that are at least reasonably wholesome. If you have a large variety from which to select, this will be to your advantage, provided you do not include too many foods at one meal. It is a good plan to get your variety from meal to meal and from day to day, but without including too many dishes at any one meal.

One of the most remarkable cases of longevity with which I have ever come in contact proved in a very pointed way the value of this suggestion. This was a woman who had lived to be over eighty years of age. During the last forty years of her life she was as agile, as clear-headed and as capable as a young woman in the heyday of her youth. I am satisfied that to a large extent the unusual vitality possessed by this woman was due to her habit of eating but one article of food two meals each day, although occasionally she would eat only one. Her meals were taken irregularly, because she would eat only when she was hungry. When she had a definite appetite it would nearly always indicate to her the particular food that she wanted. She would then prepare a meal of this food and thoroughly satisfy her appetite with it. Nothing else was eaten at that meal. This woman naturally went through some very severe trials before she adopted this diet-indeed, a terrible lesson of some sort seems necessary to compel one to follow a strict dietetic regimen. At the age of forty she was a physical wreck, having been for years tortured with rheumatism. Having vainly tried every other remedy, she finally became interested in diet, and through it finally overcame her difficulty. It might also be of interest in this connection to know that she never used salt, pepper, or condiments of any sort with her meals, and it would be well to emphasize that it is important to avoid the too free use of condiments and stimulating foods. We have used salt so long that our bodies seem adapted to it, and it is usually considered essential to the welfare of domestic stock; therefore it is a moot question as to whether it is advisable for human beings to avoid it altogether. Yet the excessive use of it to which we are prone is certainly harmful.

How is this to be avoided? If we eat our food in a hand, I have found that the longer you are without it the more you long for it, until the craving becomes much more intense than is the hunger of a man who fasts (the symptoms are those of a disease rather than of being hungry). Among the uncivilized Eskimos the dislike of salt is so strong that a saltiness imperceptible to me would prevent them from eating at all. This fact was often useful to me, and when our Eskimo visitors threatened to eat us out of house and home we could put in a little pinch of salt, and thus husband our resources without seeming inhospitable. A man who tasted anything salty at our table would quickly bethink him that he had plenty of more palatable fare in his own house. On the score of what to eat I would reiterate what I have said about the use of foods in their natural condition. The refinement of various foods has made them entirely unfit for human consumption. Of first importance without doubt is the use of the whole grain of the wheat for flour. Wheat, as produced by the Almighty, is practically a perfect food, containing all the elements required by the human body and in a proportion not very far from that found in the body. In modern methods of milling, however, the effort is made to eliminate everything in the wheat grain except the pure starch, which naturally makes a fine, smooth, white flour. The miller is not absolutely successful in his endeavor, but he does succeed in robbing the product of the natural state, that is in an uncooked form, salt can be more easily avoided, but cooking in many instances modifies the flavor to such an extent that salt seems necessary. I am not prepared to admit that it is a necessity, for I know of many who avoid the use of salt altogether and who have maintained unusual vital vigor. I have known of others, however, who have tried to eliminate salt from their diet and the results have been unsatisfactory. We may therefore say that in most cases the moderate use of salt can be recommended.

One of the most interesting expressions of opinion on the subject of salt that I have seen was a statement by Stefanson, the Arctic explorer, in his "My Quest in the Arctic," in which he discusses the diet of the Eskimos and their constitutional aversion to salt.

"Most people are in the habit of looking upon the articles of our customary diet, and especially upon salt, as necessities. We have not found them so. The longer you go without green foods and vegetables the less you long for them. Salt I have found to behave like a narcotic poison; in other words, it is as hard to break off its use as it is hard to stop the use of tobacco. But after you have been a month or so without salt you cease to long for it, and after six months I have found the taste of meat boiled in salt water positively disagreeable. In the case of such a necessary element of food as fat on the other hand, I have found that the longer you are without it the more you long for it, until the craving becomes much more intense than is the hunger of a man who fasts (the symptoms are those of a disease rather than of being hungry). Among the uncivilized Eskimos the dislike of salt is so strong that a saltiness imperceptible to me would prevent them from eating at all. This fact was often useful to me, and when our Eskimo visitors threatened to eat us out of house and home we could put in a little pinch of salt, and thus husband our resources without seeming inhospitable. A man who tasted anything salty at our table would quickly bethink him that he had plenty of more palatable fare in his own house."

On the score of what to eat I would reiterate what I have said about the use of foods in their natural condition. The refinement of various foods has made them entirely unfit for human consumption. Of first importance without doubt is the use of the whole grain of the wheat for flour. Wheat, as produced by the Almighty, is practically a perfect food, containing all the elements required by the human body and in a proportion not very far from that found in the body. In modern methods of milling, however, the effort is made to eliminate everything in the wheat grain except the pure starch, which naturally makes a fine, smooth, white flour. The miller is not absolutely successful in his endeavor, but he does succeed in robbing the product of the larger part of its food value, until it is absolutely incapable of sustaining life, and this serious mistake is without question the prime cause of the prevalence of constipation. The refining of rice by removing the coating, which contains organic salts, is another process by which is produced a food that is almost pure starch. The disease beriberi is now recognized as being due to a diet of polished rice. Where the natural unpolished rice is used this disease is both prevented and cured. In refining our sugar a similar denaturing process 'is carried on. The same is true in the grinding of corn, and in preparing a whole host of other foods. The practice of "refining" is the great food crime of the age. In addition to this the average housewife adds to our difficulties when preparing vegetables and other foods, by "draining" off the water in which they are cooked, thus throwing away the invaluable mineral elements which have been dissolved in the liquor during the process of cooking. The ultimate result of these crimes of the manufacturer and mistakes of the cook, is that the people are to a large extent starved, as far as mineral salts are concerned, in spite of the enormous food supply and the payment of the highest prices.

Though bread is supposed to be the "staff of life," it might reasonably be termed the "staff of death" when it is made entirely from white flour and is depended upon exclusively for nourishment. It is well to point out also that bread of all kinds should be avoided in some cases of weak digestion. Under such circumstances it often irritates the lining of the stomach and intestines. When symptoms of this kind are noticed bread must not be used-more especially when made with yeast. When the bread is made without yeast and is masticated very thoroughly it may do no harm. There are instances also in which there is a Strong craving for white bread and when graham or whole-wheat bread is not appetizing. When one has an abundant variety of foods and the alimentary canal is unusually active the desire for white bread can be satisfied without harmful results. In fact when the diet is varied by numerous articles of food at one meal considerable white bread can be used if it is appetizing. Those taking the treatment for constipation recommended in this book often stimulate the alimentary canal to such an extent that graham or whole-wheat products are slightly irritating in their effect. As long as such symptoms exist white bread can be used. Remember, however, that whenever there is the slightest sign of constipation white flour products of all kinds should immediately be eliminated from the diet.

As nearly as possible foods should be used in their natural condition. Those that can be enjoyed when uncooked are more valuable when eaten without cooking. When cooking is necessary the food should be cooked in such a way that there is no waste nor loss of the natural elements. Steaming and baking are both preferable in many cases to boiling; cooking in a double boiler may be especially recommended in the case of vegetables, as these are in such a case cooked in their own juices. Therefore my most important suggestions on what to eat would be: first, to select only natural foods; and second, to avoid too much variety at one meal. As to what sort of a diet one should adopt, I might say that the proper answer to a question of this kind depends largely upon one's individual condition and requirements.

Unquestionably a perfect diet is furnished by nuts and fruits. From a theoretical standpoint this would appear to be ideal. I would say, however, that very few persons can be thoroughly nourished on a limited diet of this sort, and therefore it cannot be universally recommended.

Perhaps the next diet that closely approximates perfection would be a raw or uncooked diet. This would include all the foods that can be made palatable without cooking, such as nuts and fruits of all kinds, vegetable salads, cereals and dairy products. A diet of this sort can be continued indefinitely in some cases, and where one can be thoroughly nourished on this regimen it can be highly recommended. Foods in their raw state possess a tremendous amount of vitality-building elements. They are live foods, consequently they give one life, energy, vivacity. One can usually fast longer with a smaller loss of weight and energy after a raw than after a cooked diet. But in many instances this diet does not maintain the weight and the bodily energies at high-water mark; consequently in such cases it often proves unsatisfactory, even where its first effects are pleasing to an unusual degree.

Nearly all restrictive diets are valuable for a short period where there is evidence of overeating. On this account many enthusiasts who adopt a restricted diet and who note their improved appearance and general increase of energy for a time, will be profoundly impressed with the idea that at last they have found a perfect diet. On account of their enthusiasm they will often continue such a strict dietetic regimen until it is productive of seriously harmful results. It should be kept in mind that any diet which is really adequate for all requirements will maintain your normal weight and your energy. In other words, you should feel well and look well, if your diet is as it should be. This is an invariable test, and can be depended upon absolutely.

Probably the next diet that can be recommended in many cases would be a meatless or vegetarian diet. There is absolutely no question as to the superiority of this plan over a regimen that includes meat, provided again that you can be fully nourished and that you feel energetic and capable. A vegetarian diet will usually make a better quality of tissue; you will have more endurance, and there is but little doubt that a healthy vegetarian will outlive a meat-eater, since his vital organs remain in a healthier condition for a longer period than those of one accustomed to a free use of meat.

We must admit, however, that many cannot maintain their weight and keep their full allowance of energy on a vegetarian diet. Where you find a vegetarian whose skin is white, whose lips are colorless, who is thin and seemingly in need of nourishment, you can rest assured that the diet is not agreeing with him. Such persons in virtually every instance need animal food of some sort. It is therefore wise, if you are searching for a diet that is capable of developing in you the greatest degree of mental and physical efficiency, to make a careful study of your individual condition and requirements. After you have acquired sufficient knowledge on the subject it might even be well to do some experimenting, and in that way determine what particular diet is best suited to your needs.

It is extremely difficult, however, for one to adopt a regimen which is radically different from that of those with whom he associates. You may have sufficient enthusiasm for a time to subsist on a nut-and-fruit diet or on an uncooked diet, but when your own family and friends are using other foods at all times the temptation to vary your own diet is sometimes too strong to resist, consequently you will be inclined gradually to resume the general regimen of those with whom you live.

One can, however, maintain good health without being what might be termed a dietetic crank. To be sure, where one is suffering from a disease or is definitely in need of some special diet in order to secure certain results, a very rigid diet is of great importance and should be adhered to strictly. After such results have been achieved, however, and after normal health is regained, you can secure at almost any well supplied table a selection of foods which will furnish satisfactory nourishment.

Some intelligence in selection, however, is necessary. There are a few articles of food that it would always be well to avoid. For instance, nearly all white-flour products are to be condemned. This means not only bread but biscuits, cakes, crackers, and pastries made of white flour. Unquestionably, if one is using meat freely, white-flour products are not nearly so harmful as when taken with a vegetarian diet. The meat supplies some of the deficiencies, though not all. At one time I had an experiment made which proved in a striking manner the defective character of white flour as a food. The subject tested the results of a fast of two weeks. He weighed himself before and after the fast and several times during its progress. He accurately determined his strength at all times, before, during, and at the completion of the fast. A considerable time thereafter he experimented with a diet of white-flour products for the same period of two weeks, eating white flour as commonly prepared, in the form of bread, cakes, etc. The result showed that he lost more weight and more strength while following the white-flour regimen than he had while fasting absolutely. This would seem to indicate that, in this case, at least, white-flour products were not a food, but a slow-acting poison.

Among foods especially valuable I would call attention to green salads. If possible one should eat some food of this kind each day, more especially during warm weather. They are of great value as blood purifiers and they supply to a very large extent the mineral salts. Various combinations can be used in the form of salads, and the most satisfactory dressing is probably a combination of olive oil and lemon juice. I do not recommend vinegar partly because it is seldom pure, and one never can tell what combination of chemicals it contains. Lemon juice is preferable even to the best vinegar for the purpose of salad dressing. Celery, lettuce, tomatoes, onions, water-cress, parsley, cucumbers, and other foods of this character are suitable for salad purposes. Spinach, dandelion leaves, and other greens can be recommended in their cooked form, and it is unnecessary to add that virtually all cooked vegetables are of value.

Fruits of all kinds can be recommended for the same reasons that make the green salads so useful to the body. They are of the very greatest value where there is any tendency toward biliousness. In many cases of this kind where it is undesirable to undertake an absolute fast as a means of setting the stomach right and where there is a lack of appetite, a fruit fast can be highly recommended. This is simply an exclusive diet of fresh acid fruits, such as oranges, grapefruit, grapes, cherries, apples and other fresh fruits in season. It is especially important to know in such a case that these fruits should be eaten in their strictly natural condition, properly ripened and without the addition of sugar. As a general thing a sufficient allowance of fruit and green salads will so balance the diet that one is not likely to have any trouble even if he eats heartily of the foods served at the ordinary table.

It would be well also to remember that acid fruits have valuable antiseptic (cleansing) qualities. They keep the mouth and teeth as well as the alimentary canal in a wholesome state. In fact the frequent use of acid fruit, more especially the orange, is of great value in counteracting the effects of digestive difficulties on the mouth and teeth. If a small piece of orange is taken whenever there is an unpleasant taste in the mouth it will destroy the germ life that is being rapidly propagated under such circumstances, though such symptoms indicate also the need of acid fruit of some sort by the stomach. Especially is this required if there is a craving for fruit of this sort. In such cases the rule against eating between meals may be disregarded. Whenever you have a strong desire for acid fruits between meals you are usually safe in using them. In fact they are often sorely needed under such circumstances to assist in digesting a meal that may have been eaten some hours previously. Indigestion which leaves the mouth with a foul, unpleasant taste is often noticed on awakening at night after a hearty meal the evening before. On such occasions a few swallows of water, or whatever is needed to satisfy thirst, and a small quantity of acid fruit, like the orange, are of great value. They should be well mixed and moved about in the mouth until the acid comes in contact with every part of the mouth and teeth.

When there is the slightest sign of digestive difficulties I would advise that each meal be completed with a small quantity of fruit. If you stop your meal at a time when you can enjoy the taste of acid fruit it is usually a definite proof that you have not overeaten.

Remember too that the orange, lemon and any fruit with a strong acid flavor is a splendid tooth or mouth wash, and it need not be ejected as an ordinary wash. It can be enjoyed and swallowed after mouth and teeth have been cleansed. Therefore the frequent use of oranges as a dentifrice is a habit of great value. Use them on retiring and on rising and the results will be unusually pleasing.

What foods can be used as substitutes for meat? This is a question that assumes considerable importance to those desirous of testing the vegetarian diet. I may say that almost any food that is wholesome and hearty in character and which is craved by your appetite will make a satisfactory meat substitute. Those containing a large percentage of protein are particularly desirable for this purpose. The following list will give one a general idea as to the nature of these foods: Cereals of all kinds, either in the whole grain or in the form of flaked grain, contain a fair percentage of protein and may be recommended for the purpose, although refined flour or polished grains are of no value in this way. Bread made from the whole wheat or any of the whole grains may be recommended. The "war bread" used in Europe since the outbreak of the great war is of this type. The pumpernickel and "black breads" used in various parts of Europe are so valuable from a nutritive standpoint that one can live on them entirely. Many of the farming and peasant classes of Europe live almost exclusively on breads of this type.

Nearly all the prepared foods ordinarily referred to as breakfast foods, and which are made up of whole grains of wheat, corn, oats or barley would come under this class. No breakfast food made of only a part of the wheat would be recommended for this purpose.

All kinds of beans are splendid meat substitutes, including navy beans, lima beans and kidney beans. They are what one may call hearty foods and as a rule one should lead a fairly active life to enjoy and digest them satisfactorily. The same may be said of dried peas. Lentils belong in the same class and are very similar to the bean in its nourishing elements. Beans, peas and lentils form a class known as the legumes, and contain a high percentage of protein.

Nuts of all kinds make splendid meat substitutes, though they may sometimes be found rich for a weak stomach. They need to be used in small quantities and should be eaten only at meal-time. Peanuts really belong to the legume family, but are quite as good as any kind of nuts. The only mistake in their use lies in the habit of eating them between meals. Peanut butter and nut butters are of value. When nuts are easily digested they are satisfactory in every way.

Perhaps the most popular meat substitute is the egg. Do not, however, entertain the idea that you are not eating any meat products when eggs are included in your diet. Eggs must be classed as animal food, but they are very nourishing. They contain a good supply of lime, sulphur, iron, phosphorus and other mineral salts in addition to their protein and fats. It may also be said that milk should be classed as animal food, though it is of special value from a nutritive standpoint. Milk, cheese and other milk products naturally make good substitutes for meat. Butter is a practically pure fat and will not take the place of meat in supplying protein, although it will take the place of the fatty portions of the meat. Cheese is often appropriately placed at the last part of the meal, and the statement that it will to a certain extent help to digest a hearty meal if but a small quantity is taken has been proven accurate in numerous cases.

As a milk product buttermilk may be particularly recommended as a meat substitute if one uses a considerable quantity of it. We should distinguish, however, between real buttermilk and the fermented milk or sour milk which is often sold in cities under the name of buttermilk. Fermented milk is highly recommended for all food purposes and is undoubtedly conducive to health, but from the standpoint of nutrition it has practically the same value as fresh milk. The true buttermilk, however, from which the fat-forming elements have been extracted in the form of butter, is a more purely protein product. If you use sufficient buttermilk, that is to say, two quarts or more a day, you can rest assured that you will not crave meat.

CHAPTER XIV:
Foods in the Cure of Chronic Constipation

Constipation is probably the beginning of nearly all human ailments. There are a few exceptions but not many. It is a tremendous foe to vitality. Pure blood is absolutely impossible when one is suffering from this complaint. Active functioning of the alimentary canal is absolutely essential if the blood stream is to contain those elements essential to superior vital vigor. The regimen which I suggested in the chapter on Cleansing and Stimulating the Alimentary Canal will undoubtedly be sufficient to overcome any trouble of this character provided there are not dietetic causes that are serious in nature. Where the disorder is chronic, and especially when it has extended over a term of many years, a comprehensive dietetic regimen may be necessary in addition to the adoption of measures previously suggested.

The direct cause of constipation is a relaxed and weakened condition of the muscular walls of the stomach and intestines. A certain degree of strength of these muscular structures is essential properly to facilitate digestion, assimilation and elimination. The lack of tone in these muscles is chiefly due in nearly all cases to what might be termed a concentrated diet. Our foods have been too much refined. As previously stated they are not eaten as they were created, but have been put through a prolonged milling process or other method of preparation which not only eliminates many elements of nourishment but also breaks up the food into the most minute particles, thus eliminating the rough, coarse and fibrous material in the food which ordinarily arouses what is known as the peristaltic activity of the bowels. Our methods of food preparation also materially lessen the necessity for prolonged and thorough mastication. The habit of hurriedly swallowing our food undoubtedly lessens its vitality-building possibilities, besides materially affecting the strength and general hardiness of the teeth.

Constipation is also caused in numerous instances by a lack of liquids. Men and women do not use sufficient water. One frequently loses what might be termed the water-drinking habit, usually as a result of sedentary occupations. The method of remedying constipation referred to in Chapter VI pointedly illustrates the amazing value of water in remedying conditions of this kind. It is well, however, to remember the necessity for using at least a reasonable quantity of water throughout the entire day. If you do not drink water quite freely between meals then it is advisable and actually necessary to use a certain quantity with your meals. Those who drink tea and coffee freely seem to recognize the need of this instinctively. The choice of these beverages, however, is distinctly bad. Tea and coffee are destructive to both nerves and health, but aside from these stimulating drinks one can use almost any wholesome beverage at meal-time in order to supply his cravings in this direction. Fruit drinks are excellent. I have referred to this question in a previous chapter.

Diet naturally has a tremendous influence on alimentary activity. White bread and white-flour products constitute the most serious cause of constipation. This defective food is lacking in the elements necessary to give life and vitality to the body, because the valuable covering of the grain has been removed in the milling process, while the life germ of the wheat has also been eliminated. The bran, which consists of several minute layers covering the wheat berry, has a distinct value in stimulating peristaltic action, and when it is removed, the resulting white flour must be a defective food. One of the first dietetic changes required in remedying constipation, therefore, is to eliminate white-flour products from the diet. Graham bread, or that made from the whole wheat, or any of the whole grains, rye, oats, barley, corn, is a satisfactory article of diet, and will often remedy constipation without resort to any other dietetic change.

What might be termed waste products, or fibrous material in food, are found especially valuable in promoting digestion and active functioning of the bowels. The woody fiber found in vegetables is most valuable. It is sometimes suggested that one should simply consume the juice of his foods but not the pulp. This pulp or fibrous matter, however, is especially important. Following this requirement of bulk or waste in our food, we find such remedies as sand, refined coal oil, a mineral product that passes through the alimentary canal without change, and ordinary black dirt, which is usually taken in its dried form. When using sand, it should be sterilized, and the grains should be rounded and worn smooth by the action of waves or running water. Do not use that in which the grains are sharp-edged. One or more of these products are valuable as a laxative and the devitalizing after-effects of a drug cathartic will be absent. They are, however, not by any means as pleasant as food laxatives, and remedies of this sort should not be employed except as a temporary expedient.

Whole grains of various kinds, wheat, rye, oats and barley, simmered in hot water for a long time until properly softened, not only afford a high degree of nourishment, but will be found of special value as a means of remedying constipation. They are best if used in their natural state, just as they come from the farm. They are more valuable when eaten raw with fruit or cream, or in some other palatable form, than when cooked. When flaked or crushed, as in the case of ordinary oatmeal, they may be used with figs, dates, raisins and a little cream, or they may be eaten with a little honey. One bowl of this class of food, either raw or cooked, each day, is very effective in overcoming constipation. Salads of various kinds not only have great value by way of supplying food for the nerves, but they are also worth while for their mild laxative effect. I would recommend all forms of uncooked green food, chiefly to be used in the form of salads, such as lettuce, tomatoes, onions, celery, radishes, cucumbers, cold slaw, water-cress, parsley, and the like. All cooked green vegetables such as spinach, asparagus, string beans, fresh green peas, Brussels sprouts, dandelion leaves, greens, cabbages, mushrooms and other foods of this sort will likewise be helpful.

Fruits are of even greater value for their laxative qualities. One should use them freely for ordinary health building, but especially when suffering from this complaint. Apples, oranges, grapefruit, peaches, plums, grapes, and various berries are exceptionally good for increasing alimentary activity, though all kinds of fruit are valuable. Prunes and figs are particularly recommended. Such acid fruits as lemons, oranges and grapefruit are valuable not only for their stimulating qualities in connection with constipation, but also because of their antiseptic influence.

Cheese is very constipating to those inclined in this direction. All forms of cheese and food combinations containing it should be avoided. Spaghetti and macaroni prepared in this way are especially inadvisable, though it may be said that even when served without cheese spaghetti and macaroni are constipating. Rice in the ordinary polished form, as usually sold, is practically a pure starch and should be avoided. The same applies to tapioca, sago and foods of this character. Needless to say white crackers, cookies and cakes are to be classed with white bread. One should use brown sugar in place of white wherever possible, or use the pure New Orleans molasses. It is often difficult to secure this, however, inasmuch as most of the molasses on the market is made up chiefly of glucose or corn syrup, and often contains harmful chemical preservatives. It is best to avoid sugar altogether and to use honey for all purposes of sweetening, as honey is less inclined to fermentation.

Milk in some cases is inclined to produce constipation when used in connection with the ordinary diet. An exclusive and full diet of milk, is rarely constipating except during the first few days of the diet, but when milk is added to the ordinary foods, it frequently has a tendency in this direction. Buttermilk or fermented milk can often be used to advantage if sweet milk should prove constipating to the patient.

Muscular weakness and defective circulation are prominent causes of constipation in many cases. This accounts for this disorder being found so frequently among sedentary workers. Inactivity, the cause of many ills, is particularly prominent in contributing to this trouble. Therefore muscular exercise is perhaps a most effective means of permanently remedying constipation. Exercise has a direct mechanical influence upon the entire alimentary canal. The contraction of the abdominal muscles and the bending or other movements of the trunk of the body produce a certain amount of movement in and pressure upon the digestive organs in a direct mechanical way. Walking, for instance, is of extraordinary value in remedying this difficulty because of its stimulating influence upon the entire functional system, and the slight jar of each step without doubt has a direct mechanical effect. Walking furthermore is a tremendous factor in the building of vitality and this helps indirectly in remedying constipation.

But there are also various special exercises that particularly affect the alimentary canal. Bending forward and backward and from side to side and also various twisting movements of the trunk have a special influence in this direction. They actually massage the internal organs, and this means a great deal where there is any digestive weakness or lack of activity in the bowels. What I term inner-strength exercises, or as they may also be called, pressure movements, are also of considerable value. An example of this type of exercise will be found in placing the right forearm across the stomach, grasping the right wrist with the left hand, and then with the strength of both arms pressing vigorously inward upon the stomach for a moment. Now relax and repeat. Bringing up the right knee and left knee alternately, with strong pressure, using vigorously the strength of the arms against the abdominal region, is also a good example of this type of exercise, which has proven very effective in numerous cases. Other exercises of this kind (see Chapter XV) can be applied to all parts of the upper body with great advantage to the inner organs, since such movements are of remarkable value in stimulating alimentary activity.

In line with exercise of this kind, massage and percussion treatment of the abdominal region is likewise effective. The massage should be deep and may be administered by the closed fist. A wide circular movement is advantageous for this purpose, the hand being moved in the direction of the hands of a clock, that is to say, up the right side, across, down the left side and continuing around in that manner. Rolling a baseball around in the same manner, pressing deeply though without strain, will afford an excellent form of massage for this particular purpose. The percussion treatment that I have suggested consists in alternate tapping or striking this region of the body with both hands. A chopping movement, using the outside edge of the hands, is very effective, and if you are very vigorous, the closed fist may be used. Striking repeatedly and alternately with the two fists, go over the entire region of the stomach and abdomen. This can be done gently or vigorously, according to your condition, and it is an invaluable and effective means of stimulating peristalsis and functional vigor. Mechanical vibration may also be suggested.

Cathartics are always to be condemned. The ordinary cathartic or laxative acts by reason of its irritating qualities. As a rule it abstracts the water from the intestinal walls, and the adjacent tissues, and the ultimate effect is to leave one in worse condition than before. Those who have been accustomed to the drug treatment of constipation, usually find the condition growing continuously more stubborn. Larger and larger doses of the cathartic must be taken to secure results until the function is practically paralyzed. There could be no greater mistake. If some laxative is required and sand cannot be used, the best remedy is ordinary table salt. Stir up a level teaspoonful in a glass of water and drink it. This has a mild laxative action. Or take daily two to four tablespoonfuls of ordinary bran in a glass of water. This bran may also be stirred into soups and cereals or mixed with whole-wheat flour when making bread. Olive oil also should be used freely.

As an emergency treatment, however, the enema is most satisfactory, and when employed it is best to do it thoroughly. I do not advocate the regular and continuous use of this measure. One should not come to depend upon it. A natural action is desirable, and this can invariably be brought about by a proper diet, as above suggested, by exercise and by a sufficient amount of water. The enema or colon-flushing should be used only when absolutely necessary, though in case of acute disease, where rapid purification is essential, the enema is imperatively demanded, and no household should be without an outfit for giving this treatment.

To some the continuous use of the colon-flushing treatment is inclined to be debilitating and in rare cases complaints have been made that it dilates the colon and weakens its muscular structures. This is occasionally true in the case of the hot enema. A fairly cool enema is less objectionable, while a cold enema has a decided tonic effect in contracting and strengthening the peristaltic muscles. The cold enema is less effective as a cleansing agent, as it does not have the relaxing effect of the hot enema. In most cases an enema of neutral temperature, or at about that of the body, may be suggested, though if one has been using this treatment very much it would be better to use either a cool or cold enema, if strong enough, in order to secure its contracting and tonic effect. If the cold water causes cramps one should modify the temperature.

Usually it is best to use plain water for the enema. In a case of illness where quick and radical results are required, a hot soap-suds enema may be suggested, but you should remember that this always has the effect of removing the natural oils and is inclined to leave the colon in an irritated condition. A saline solution is to be especially commended where there is a serious catarrhal condition of the intestines, or where there is much inflammation or irritation, such as might be manifested in extreme cases by bloody stools. For a normal saline solution use one teaspoonful of ordinary salt to a quart of water, or four teaspoonfuls to a four-quart enema. Glycerin is frequently suggested, but it is not to be generally recommended. If one follows these methods persistently, constipation, even in its most aggravated forms, can be overcome. In some instances almost any one of the suggestions offered will bring about the results desired, but in a chronic case one should depend not on one but on a combination of all of these various remedial measures. The improvement in the condition of your skin, in the purity of your blood, and in the degree of energy that you will enjoy will more than repay you for your efforts in following the various suggestions made for cleansing, strengthening, and vitalizing the alimentary canal.

CHAPTER XV:
Pressure Movements for Building Inner Strength

Several years ago I discovered a unique and very effective means of strengthening the heart, lungs, stomach and other internal organs. I arranged a system of lessons, consisting of various pressure movements, which I termed an Inner Strength Course. As my experience with this course had been limited, I refrained at the time from presenting its fundamental theories to the general public. I issued the course in a series of four lessons, and the strength of each applicant was ascertained through questions before the course was sent to him. The experience with several hundred students, however, has so thoroughly confirmed the value of this method of internal vitality building that I am now in a position where I can present the ideas upon which it is based to the general public. The usual price of this course was five dollars, and several thousand courses were sold at this price, each student naturally receiving a certain amount of personal attention. The same ideas, however, are presented in this chapter, with the warning that those who use the pressure exercises recommended must take care to avoid pressing upon the internal organs beyond their resisting power.

The various forms of pressure movements recommended are clearly illustrated and those who are not especially strong should begin with a very mild pressure and with the open hand placed upon the abdomen or chest, though where ordinary or unusual strength is possessed, the side of the open or closed hand could be used. These exercises are especially valuable for strengthening the heart where the pressure movements are used very freely near this particular organ. They can be highly recommended for strengthening the stomach though they should not be used immediately after a meal. I referred to their value in the chapter on constipation in connection with the treatment of this ailment. After a long trial this system of increasing the internal strength is highly recommended, and will be found of special value as a means of varying the health-building methods that may be adopted for securing throbbing vitality. They are not a necessary part of the plan of body building especially recommended in this volume, but are presented merely as a valuable means of varying your efforts in working for increased vitality.

It is an interesting fact that in some forms of athletics, the body is subjected to a certain amount of internal stimulation similar to that which I have systematized in these movements. This is especially true in wrestling, where the vital organism is often compelled to endure a great deal of pressure of this kind. The same is true of American football, although this is too violent for those who are not in an unusually vigorous condition.

To suit these varying degrees of strength I have arranged these movements so that the first series (A) is comparatively mild. Those who are not already vigorous can probably use the advanced form of treatment, but in most cases it will be best to take them up gradually. In cases of rupture, or where the abdominal region is weak, there is a possibility of injury if one makes the movements too vigorous.

The first series, however, in which the open palm of the hand is used, is quite safe in all cases, if reasonable care is used. In each of these pressure movements remember that the pressure should be applied for one moment only, and then relaxed, repeating the pressure and moving the position of the hands in accordance with the directions accompanying each photograph.

When a feeling of pain or great tenderness is noted in pressing upon any part of the body, this should be regarded as a warning that the pressure is not to be repeated. If there is only a feeling of uneasiness you can usually continue with the treatment and the discomfort will disappear in practically every instance. And while an acute sense of pain indicates the necessity for avoiding pressure on that particular part, yet it is sometimes a good plan to exert the pressure upon adjacent or surrounding parts, thereby influencing the circulation, and continuing the treatment until the inflammation which is the cause of the pain gradually disappears. One should be careful to exercise moderation in all cases, however.

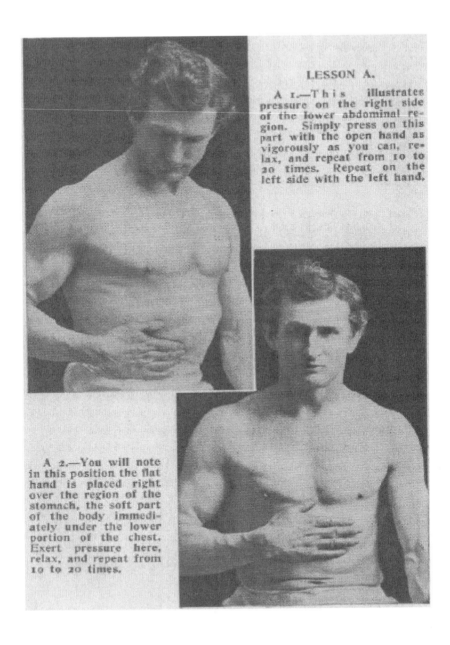

LESSON A.

A 1.—This illustrates pressure on the right side of the lower abdominal region. Simply press on this part with the open hand as vigorously as you can, relax, and repeat from 10 to 20 times. Repeat on the left side with the left hand.

A 2.—You will note in this position the flat hand is placed right over the region of the stomach, the soft part of the body immediately under the lower portion of the chest. Exert pressure here, relax, and repeat from 10 to 20 times.

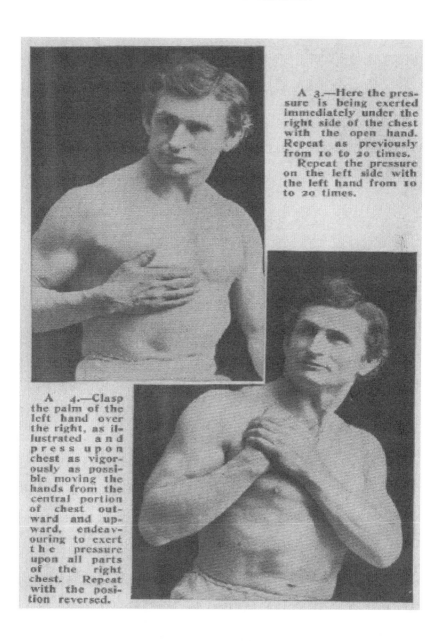

A 3.—Here the pressure is being exerted immediately under the right side of the chest with the open hand. Repeat as previously from 10 to 20 times.
Repeat the pressure on the left side with the left hand from 10 to 20 times.

A 4.—Clasp the palm of the left hand over the right, as illustrated and press upon chest as vigorously as possible moving the hands from the central portion of chest outward and upward, endeavouring to exert the pressure upon all parts of the right chest. Repeat with the position reversed.

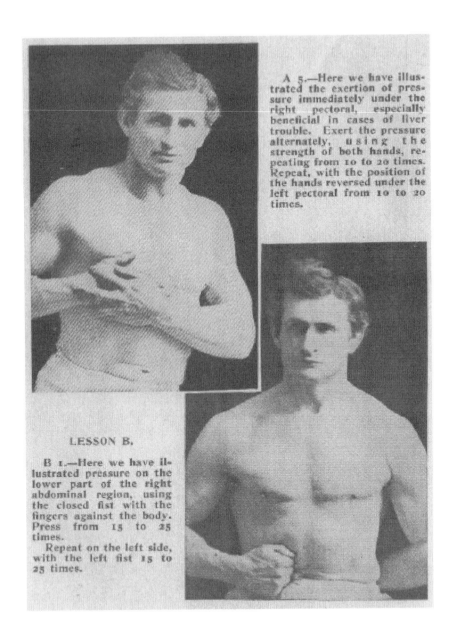

A 5.—Here we have illustrated the exertion of pressure immediately under the right pectoral, especially beneficial in cases of liver trouble. Exert the pressure alternately, using the strength of both hands, repeating from 10 to 20 times. Repeat, with the position of the hands reversed under the left pectoral from 10 to 20 times.

LESSON B.

B 1.—Here we have illustrated pressure on the lower part of the right abdominal region, using the closed fist with the fingers against the body. Press from 15 to 25 times.

Repeat on the left side, with the left fist 15 to 25 times.

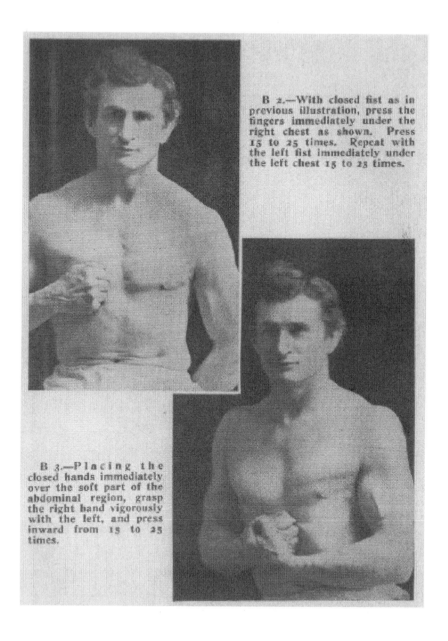

B 2.—With closed fist as in previous illustration, press the fingers immediately under the right chest as shown. Press 15 to 25 times. Repeat with the left fist immediately under the left chest 15 to 25 times.

B 3.—Placing the closed hands immediately over the soft part of the abdominal region, grasp the right hand vigorously with the left, and press inward from 15 to 25 times.

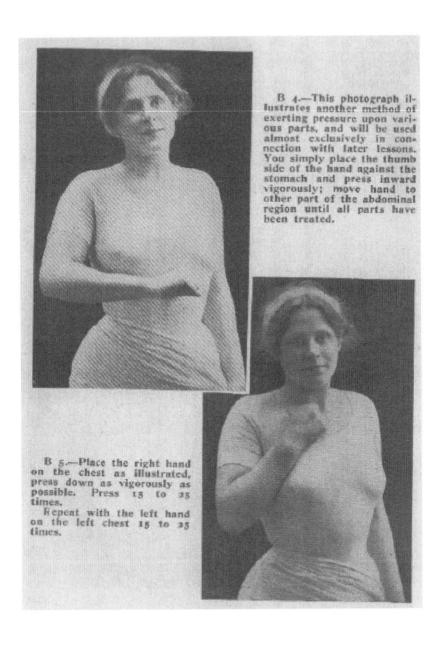

B 4.—This photograph illustrates another method of exerting pressure upon various parts, and will be used almost exclusively in connection with later lessons. You simply place the thumb side of the hand against the stomach and press inward vigorously; move hand to other part of the abdominal region until all parts have been treated.

B 5.—Place the right hand on the chest as illustrated, press down as vigorously as possible. Press 15 to 25 times.

Repeat with the left hand on the left chest 15 to 25 times.

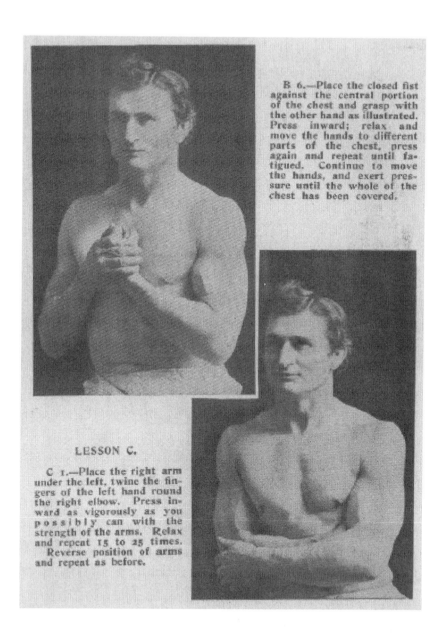

B 6.—Place the closed fist against the central portion of the chest and grasp with the other hand as illustrated. Press inward; relax and move the hands to different parts of the chest, press again and repeat until fatigued. Continue to move the hands, and exert pressure until the whole of the chest has been covered.

LESSON C.

C 1.—Place the right arm under the left, twine the fingers of the left hand round the right elbow. Press inward as vigorously as you possibly can with the strength of the arms. Relax and repeat 15 to 25 times.
Reverse position of arms and repeat as before.

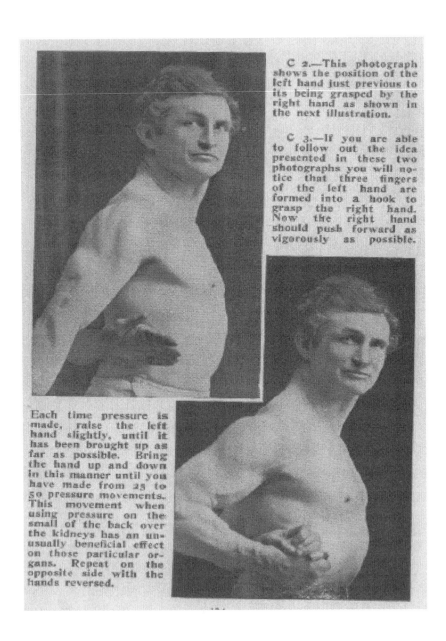

C 2.—This photograph shows the position of the left hand just previous to its being grasped by the right hand as shown in the next illustration.

C 3.—If you are able to follow out the idea presented in these two photographs you will notice that three fingers of the left hand are formed into a hook to grasp the right hand. Now the right hand should push forward as vigorously as possible.

Each time pressure is made, raise the left hand slightly, until it has been brought up as far as possible. Bring the hand up and down in this manner until you have made from 25 to 50 pressure movements. This movement when using pressure on the small of the back over the kidneys has an unusually beneficial effect on those particular organs. Repeat on the opposite side with the hands reversed.

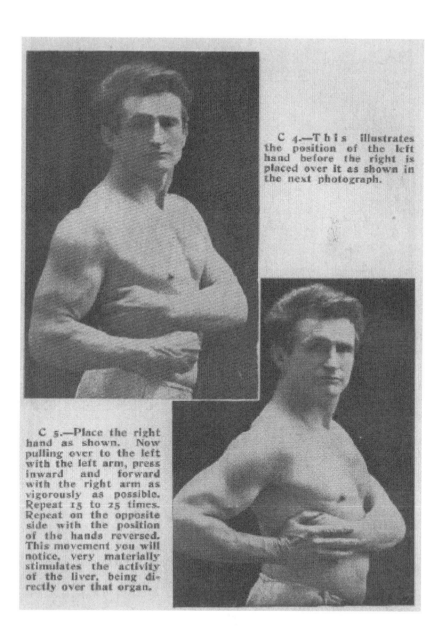

C 4.—T h i s illustrates the position of the left hand before the right is placed over it as shown in the next photograph.

C 5.—Place the right hand as shown. Now pulling over to the left with the left arm, press inward and forward with the right arm as vigorously as possible. Repeat 15 to 25 times. Repeat on the opposite side with the position of the hands reversed. This movement you will notice, very materially stimulates the activity of the liver, being directly over that organ.

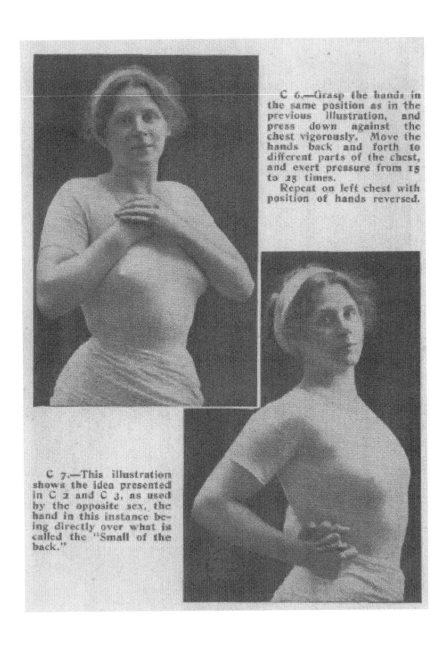

C 6.—Grasp the hands in the same position as in the previous illustration, and press down against the chest vigorously. Move the hands back and forth to different parts of the chest, and exert pressure from 15 to 25 times.

Repeat on left chest with position of hands reversed.

C 7.—This illustration shows the idea presented in C 2 and C 3, as used by the opposite sex, the hand in this instance being directly over what is called the "Small of the back."

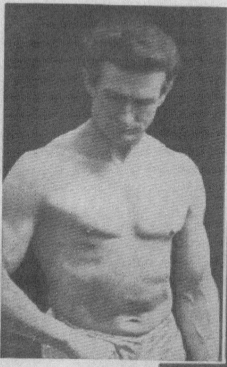

LESSON D.

D 1.—Showing the position of the right hand, ready for the left hand to grasp it, for the purpose of exerting pressure on the lower right portion of the abdominal region. When exerting pressure in each instance move the hand slightly upward until it finally reaches the lower part of the chest.

Repeat the exercise on the left side with left hand, but note that when pressing on the right side always move the right hand from the lower part of the abdomen

upward and when pressing on the left side always move the hand downward. This is especially important if there is any tendency towards constipation, for in such circumstances, pressure exerted in this way will have an unusually beneficial effect in stimulating the activity of the bowels.

D 2.—Showing how the hand is placed in the central portion of the abdominal region, ready for grasping with the other hand, as shown in the next photograph.

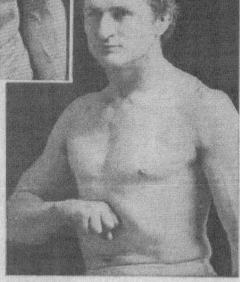

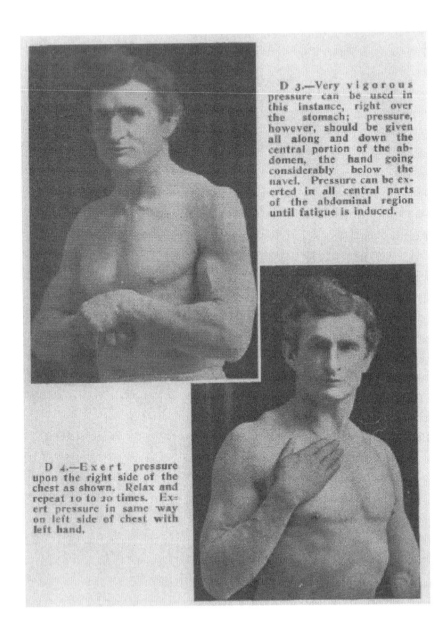

D 3.—Very vigorous pressure can be used in this instance, right over the stomach; pressure, however, should be given all along and down the central portion of the abdomen, the hand going considerably below the navel. Pressure can be exerted in all central parts of the abdominal region until fatigue is induced.

D 4.—Exert pressure upon the right side of the chest as shown. Relax and repeat 10 to 20 times. Exert pressure in same way on left side of chest with left hand.

The second series (B) in which the closed hand is used is somewhat more vigorous, and this is made still more energetic by grasping the first hand with the other so that the pressure may be applied with the strength of both the arms. As the student progresses, the number of times that pressure is applied at each part of the body may be increased, so that at the conclusion of the treatment he may feel thoroughly tired, thus showing that he is making good progress toward the goal in view.

The third series (C) includes movements especially intended for stimulating the functional regions from the back of the body, and should be given close attention. They are especially valuable for strengthening the kidneys. The last and most vigorous of the movements (series D) are especially powerful in their influence upon the organs lying within the chest as well as upon those beneath the diaphragm. The heart and lungs will be very effectually stimulated and strengthened in this way. In chronic bronchitis, coughs and colds on the lungs these movements applied to the chest will be very helpful, besides directly strengthening these parts.

You can absolutely depend upon it that when you have reached a condition in which you can exert the most vigorous pressure upon all of these parts, and do it with comfort and pleasurable results, your "department of the interior" is in a strong and healthy condition. You will find a radical change in the entire internal organism. You will find that the abdominal organs feel more solid and substantial, while the muscular walls of this region are far stronger. You will have a sense of strength in this region, and this is absolutely the case in so far as the external muscles of this part of the body are concerned. But the more valuable gain will be in the strength of the organs themselves. These organs are partly muscular in character, and they are firm and strong, or soft and flaccid, in accordance with the intelligent consideration that they receive and the amount of exercise given them.

Before long you should be able to use almost your entire strength in exerting pressure, and feel nothing but beneficial results. But when doing this it may be well to change the position of the hand slightly for each application of pressure, rather than to repeat such strenuous treatment so many times in one spot. The idea is to exert pressure throughout the entire region of the abdomen, chest, sides and back.

It may occur to the reader that this form of exercise for the vital organs has a certain distant similarity to some features of massage treatment, known as deep massage. However, this method is much more vigorous than any form of massage, and is of a character to build a degree of real internal strength that cannot be attained through massage of any kind. And it has the advantage of being convenient for self-application.

After a time you may be able to originate pressure movements of your own. One of my friends writes that he has used a similar idea associated with a vibratory motion. He slightly agitates the hand in different directions while pressing inwards. This is well worth a trial, and it partakes very much of the nature of massage. Another good practice is to inhale a deep breath and then while holding this breath apply pressure all along the central portion of the abdominal region, from the breastbone downwards, from ten to twenty times. Then, without exhaling the breath, draw in all the additional air you can and repeat the pressure movements six to twelve times, after which you may be able to take in still more air. One should be careful not to carry this holding of the breath too far. At the first signs of discomfort the breath should be exhaled quickly.

CHAPTER XVI: Blood Purification

If one could maintain his blood in absolute purity disease would be virtually impossible. The blood is the life. You are what you are through the influence of the blood that circulates throughout your entire body.

Now, a proper supply of pure blood, as previously stated, depends first of all upon proper digestion and assimilation. This involves naturally a strengthening diet with a supply of foods that contain all of the elements required by the body and which will permit of a pure and perfect condition of the blood. Next in importance are the chemical changes which take place in this life-giving fluid as it passes through the lungs. Following this, the purity of the life stream depends upon the various organs that have to do with elimination; that is to say, the throwing off from the blood of the various accumulated wastes and poisons that are inimical to life. Now you might call this the blood-purifying process. The removal of these various waste elements from the blood depends entirely upon the proper activity of the depurating organs.

I have already referred to the great importance of an active alimentary canal. You might say that the lower part of the alimentary canal is the sewer of the body. It removes a large amount of the impurities. In some cases of fasting that I have personally supervised, there has been a daily action of the bowels merely from the waste matter that has accumulated. The debris that is removed from the body in this way does not by any means consist entirely of the remains of food that is not absorbed by the circulatory system. The blood is purified to a large extent by the various waste elements that seek the alimentary canal for an outlet. If these waste products were allowed to remain in the circulation they would produce seriously injurious results. Therefore, in the general scheme of blood purification an active alimentary canal is of first importance.

I may say that proper breathing, together with the facilitation of this function through active exercise, is the next feature of importance in blood purification. Following this we can without doubt reasonably maintain that a certain amount of activity of the kidneys is desired. This will nearly always be accomplished if one drinks the amount of water which is essential to satisfy a natural thirst. Remember, however, that modern habits are often inclined partially to eliminate or entirely to destroy what one might call a natural thirst. For instance, there are various sedentary occupations in which one becomes so absorbed in his work that the desire for water will be ignored, and where this mistake is made for a long period, one acquires the habit of going without water, and consequently the natural desire is to a large extent lost. In such cases, it is even important to bring back the appetite for water. Have a glass of water at hand and take a few swallows now and then. Or, what would be better yet, carry out the suggestion which I have given in a former chapter on the drinking of hot water. That will usually supply the system with the proper amount of liquid necessary to insure normal activity of the kidneys.

The next means of blood purification is one which rarely receives a great amount of attention. I refer to the eliminative function of the skin. We have more definite control over and can more easily influence this particular channel of elimination than any other. The skin unquestionably throws off a tremendous amount of impurities. Where but little attention is given it, where one bathes at infrequent intervals and to a large extent smothers the skin with a surplus amount of clothing, the activity of the eliminative function of the skin is greatly reduced. There are various means at hand for stimulating the activity of the skin which are of unusual value in connection with blood purification.

One of the simplest methods both of improvising the texture of the skin and accelerating its functional processes is found in dry friction. This friction can be applied with the palm of the hand, with a rough towel, or with friction brushes. In order to secure the greatest advantages of a friction bath it is advisable to brush or rub the surface of every part of the body until it assumes a pinkish glow from the increased peripheral circulation induced by the friction. Where the skin is rough or covered with pimples this suggestion is of especial value. When using friction brushes for this purpose one should not attempt to use very stiff brushes in the beginning, for they will scratch too much. Soft, fair skins usually cannot stand such rough treatment as well as can a thicker skin, or one which is oily in character. In many cases a dry Turkish bath towel will answer the purpose splendidly. If the skin is rather tender it suffices to use the palms of both hands. After becoming accustomed to the friction, however, you will find that you will be able to enjoy stiffer brushes and I would suggest using a fairly stiff brush so long as it is not too uncomfortable. You will find that as you become accustomed to the treatment the skin will become softer and smoother as a result. Also it will become more active. This dry friction bath may be taken each morning following your exercises. If you take a cold bath it should follow the friction. First exercise, then employ the friction rub, and then bathe. I would suggest that from five to ten minutes at least be devoted to this friction. It will furnish some exercise in connection with the rubbing, will quicken the general circulation, and will give you that warmth of body which makes the cold bath desirable and delightful.

Air baths are likewise valuable as a means of promoting activity in the eliminative function of the skin. Primitive man, living in a state of Nature, was not burdened with clothing. There was nothing to interfere with the healthy activity of his epidermis. There can be no question that the smothering of the skin by our clothing has much to do with defective elimination of wastes, and the more nearly we can avoid clothing, or the less clothing we can wear, the better. When possible, therefore, and especially in warm weather, it is advisable to remove all clothing and let the air come in contact with the surface of the body. This not only has a pronounced effect upon the purification of the blood but it likewise has a tonic effect upon the nervous system. In the same way the friction rub has a stimulating effect upon the nerves. This is due to the fact that in the skin are located a million or more of tiny nerve endings or so-called "end organs" of the nerves. These peripheral nerve endings are naturally influenced by all conditions that affect the skin, whether in the form of friction, air baths, cold baths, or baths of other temperatures. The air bath, therefore, has a splendid tonic effect and may be particularly recommended for those suffering with "nerves."

Sun baths are especially effective as a means of stimulating activity of the skin, and promoting elimination. Sun baths likewise have a very powerful influence upon the entire organism inasmuch as they stimulate metabolism or cell-activity. They directly affect the circulation and promote the formation of red corpuscles. The sun is the center of all energy and life upon this earth. It is our great vitalizing and life-giving principle, both in the realms of animal life and plant life. It is only natural, therefore, that sun baths should have a profound influence upon the body.

A word of caution, however, is required because of the tremendous power of the sun and its powerful chemical effect when sun bathing is carried too far. Those of very fair skins particularly need to be careful. Brunettes, with considerable pigment of the skin can stand a great deal of sunlight without harm, but light-skinned persons, while needing a certain amount of sunlight, should not expose themselves for too long a time to the midday sun in summer, or at least not until they have gradually become sufficiently tanned to do so. Everyone knows the painful character of a sunburn. This only illustrates the powerful chemical effect of the sun's rays. In taking sun baths one should very gradually accustom himself to the sunshine until he is so tanned that the pigment in his skin will protect him. The short or chemical rays of the sun are actually destructive to white men in the tropics. In May, June and July they have a pronounced chemical effect even in our own latitude. They are stimulating up to a certain point, but beyond that point one should be careful. I may say, therefore, that brunettes in summer may take sun baths even at noon, but blondes should take them preferably before nine or ten o'clock in the morning or after three o'clock in the afternoon. In winter, however, when the sun's rays are more slanting, the sun baths can be taken even by the blondes at any time. And because of the more limited amount of sunlight in winter, special attention should be given to sun bathing during that season.

Everyone needs a certain amount of sunlight, and if you cannot take a sun bath regularly every day you should at least wear clothing of a character that will permit the light-rays of the sun to penetrate. I will refer to this again, however, in the chapter on the subject of clothing.

After all that we can say in regard to these various methods of stimulating the skin there is really nothing so effective as active exercise for those who are strong enough to take a sufficient amount of it. Exercise, so far as function of the skin is concerned, is valuable because of the copious perspiration which is induced when one gets enough of it. In these days great numbers of people no longer "earn their bread by the sweat of their brow," and their health suffers in consequence. If you do not have to perform such an amount of physical labor as will promote free perspiration, then for the sake of acquiring the very purest quality of blood your special exercise should be sufficiently active and continuous to bring about free perspiration. There is really nothing so effective as a good old-fashioned "sweat" for rapidly purifying the blood. Anyone who perspires each and every day as a result of physical activity, and whose habits are fairly satisfactory in other respects, can depend upon enjoying absolutely pure blood, or a condition which is not far from it.

It does not matter what form of physical activity is employed to bring about this result. It may take the form of work that is useful and productive in character, or it may be play that is sufficiently active to cause deep, free breathing and bring out the perspiration. For those who are vigorous enough, cross-country running, wrestling, boxing, tennis and other games which involve real muscular effort continued for some time, will all prove satisfactory for this purpose. If you are anxious to purify your blood in cold weather it might be well to wear a good heavy sweater while taking such exercise in order to maintain a marked degree of warmth and thus bring out the perspiration in plentiful quantities. It is always well to avoid becoming chilled too quickly after exercise of this kind.

It is not alone in stimulating the eliminative function of the skin that exercise has a blood-purifying effect; it accelerates all the functions of the body, it stimulates greater activity of the lungs and of the kidneys. It promotes such an active circulation through all the minute structures of the body that accumulations of waste and dead matter are taken up and swept on to be thrown out through the natural channels of elimination. Under conditions of physical stagnation, when the circulation is less active, much of this waste matter tends to remain in the tissues of the body, accumulating and interfering with cell activity and normal functioning in general. The vigorous circulation of the blood induced by exercise gradually has the effect of flushing out all of the bodily tissues, and in that way has an internal cleansing effect that cannot be attained by any other means. In another chapter I have referred to the powerful influence of the drinking of hot water in connection with exercise as a means of promoting a more free circulation, but exercise under any circumstances tends to the same result, and for this reason as well as because of the perspiration brought about, exercise must be regarded as perhaps the most important of all measures for blood purification. No man can be continuously healthy without exercise. No man or woman can be internally clean, in the strictest sense, without a proper amount of daily exercise.

However, for those who are not strong enough to take a large amount of exercise, and who cannot in this way bring about free perspiration, other methods of accelerating the activity of the pores of the skin may be employed. I have already referred to the influence of air baths, friction baths and sun baths. Remember that through these agencies the pores may be made very active without any apparent result in the form of liquid perspiration, for under ordinary conditions perspiration evaporates and the body may not become wet. It is only when one perspires very rapidly that perspiration is manifested in the moistening of the skin. When taking your air baths there may be marked activity of the skin without any appearance of "sweat."

Various forms of bathing have the effect of inducing rapid elimination. Russian and Turkish baths are commonly used for this purpose, and every "man about town" knows the value of Russian and Turkish baths as a means of clearing his system and even of "clearing his head" through the profuse perspiration induced by the treatment. There is no question that these baths are effective in this direction, though it may be said that they are only a poor substitute for daily exercise as a blood-purifying measure. The man who neglects his requirements in the way of physical activity may strive to make up for it by a Turkish bath, but cannot get the same results, although it is true he can accomplish a great deal in this way. The great objection to Turkish and Russian bath establishments is to be found in the unsatisfactory ventilation usual in such places.

As a rule the Russian or vapor bath is to be preferred to the Turkish, or dry, hot air. Especially if one is not very strong the steam bath is preferable. If one is vigorous, however, and has a strong heart, the dry hot air room will be very effective. Naturally the "rubbing" and other adjunctive treatment in the Turkish bath establishment are all beneficial.

The influence of these measures (the Russian and Turkish baths) in purifying the blood may be secured at home through the agency of other baths. A cabinet bath in the home will be equally effective in providing either a steam bath or a dry, hot-air bath. Naturally, a shower, or at least a quick sponging with cold water, should follow all such baths. If there is no bath cabinet in the home beneficial results can be secured by means of a hot-water bath. Hot water has a profound influence upon the elimination of wastes and impurities through the skin. In cases of kidney disease, where the kidneys are unable to perform their work, it is often possible to keep one alive by making the skin do the work of the kidneys through frequent hot baths. The tub should be filled with hot water at a temperature of from 105 up to 112 or 115 degrees Fahrenheit, that is to say, as hot as it can be endured, and one should remain in this bath from ten to twenty minutes, or as long as one's condition will permit. It may be a good plan to get into the water at a lower temperature, for instance, starting with water at 102 to 104 degrees, then afterwards adding hot water so as to raise the temperature to 108 or 112 degrees, or even higher. It is really necessary to use a bath thermometer (they can be obtained at a cost of ten or fifteen cents in any drug store) to regulate the temperature of the water. Sufferers from any derangement of the heart or those handicapped by serious vital depletion should not use the water too hot. In such cases it may be well to limit the temperature to 103 to 105 degrees and to limit the duration of the bath to five or ten minutes. In such cases it will be necessary to take the bath more frequently, perhaps each evening, in order to secure results in the way of active elimination. If one is strong enough, however, and merely wishes to purify the blood one may be able to stay in the water from twenty to thirty minutes and to raise the temperature of the bath to 115 degrees or more. The hot bath is much used in Japan and the natives there almost parboil themselves, using water at a temperature as high as 120 degrees. But it is not necessary to go to such extremes. It is most important that one should leave the bath immediately upon feeling any sense of weakness, dizziness or discomfort of any sort. If you feel oppressed by a sense of overheating, do not linger in the water but get out of it immediately. You will usually find that your face will perspire freely within a few minutes after being in the bath. This indicates its rapid eliminative effect. Such a bath will not accomplish exactly the same work as a cabinet or Turkish bath, but good results can be secured therefrom. The hot bath when used for perspiration purposes should be followed by a quick sponging with cold water or by a cold shower. An excellent plan is to have conveniently at hand what is called a hand spray, attached to a long rubber tube. By attaching this to the faucet and turning on the cold water one may quickly spray all parts of the body while standing in the tub of hot water. Finally, the feet may be sprayed with cold water on getting out of the tub. Rub dry quickly and thoroughly with a rough towel, after which wrap up warmly so that you may continue to perspire. It is most essential that one should not cool off too quickly and certainly that one should not become chilled after a bath of this sort. This hot bath is rather strenuous treatment, but it is effective, if one is strong vitally, for rapidly purifying the blood and eliminating the poisons in the body in any toxemic condition. It will be found valuable in the case of grippe or of a bad cold, in syphilis, or in any other disease characterized by a poisoned condition of the system and in which there is no fever present. In the case of fever, which also invariably involves a toxemic condition of the body, the elimination of the poisons through the skin should be accomplished by methods which do not involve the external use of heat in this manner.

Wet-sheet packs, both of the entire body and of parts of the body, are among the most effective of rapid blood-purifying measures. Frequently where one is confined to bed a hot-blanket pack will answer the same purpose as the hot bath just described. Where there is high fever a cold wet-sheet pack may be employed. This will relieve the high temperature to a marked extent, and will also eliminate the poisons of the body in a most remarkable way. The sheet pack is applied by first wringing one or two sheets out of cold water and then wrapping them completely around the naked patient, with the exception of the head. If a single sheet is used the flap on one side may be wrapped around the body under the arms and the flap from the other side passed over the outside of the arms. The patient should then be wrapped up thoroughly with warm blankets, fastened with safety pins.

He will quickly react with warmth, although if the vitality is low it may be well to place hot irons at the feet to insure quick recuperation with warmth. One may remain in such a pack for two or three hours, or if it is applied in the evening one may remain in it all night, provided sleep follows and no discomfort is noticed.

Where the recuperative powers are weak a wet-sheet pack which covers the entire body, may tax the vitality too much and under such circumstances a chest and abdominal pack may be used. This is really a partial sheet pack covering the trunk of the body from the hips and abdomen to the line running round the chest just under the arms. A hot pack of this kind is in itself very effective, although where there is fever the pack should be applied cold. In all such packs it is well to lay several blankets on your couch first, then quickly place the wet sheet upon it so that after the sheet has been wrapped around the body the sides of the blanket can be pulled over so as completely to envelop the patient.

These methods are all suggested because of their effectiveness in stimulating the activity of the skin where one is not able to bring this about through exercise and perspiration. In all chronic conditions, however, in which it is essential to purify the blood, the daily practice of dry friction or air baths is particularly advised. Do not overlook the value of the hot-water-drinking regimen in combination with exercise, which I offered in the chapter on Cleansing and Stimulating the Alimentary Canal. It is especially important to guard against constipation if there is any tendency in that direction, and above all things, daily muscular activity is absolutely essential. Inasmuch as many foods have great value in the purification of the blood, I have referred to this particular aspect of the question in the chapter on What to Eat.

Before leaving this subject it should be said that where there is any necessity for a rapid, thorough and effective cleansing of the entire system there is nothing that will accomplish this result as effectually as fasting. Fasting is the greatest of all methods of purification. Where there is any derangement of the system, with temporary loss of appetite, it is usually advisable to fast until the appetite returns and a short fast of from one to three days is usually sufficient. Where there is any serious disorder and it is necessary to undergo an extensive course of blood purification a prolonged fast of many days or even several weeks may be required. Fasting is such an important subject in itself that I can-. not give any detailed suggestions in regard to it in this volume. Before fasting one should make a comprehensive study of its physical effects and especially should one be informed on proper methods of breaking a fast.

During a fast all of the eliminative functions of the body are exceedingly active. If there is any surplus material the body consumes it during the fast. Owing to the complete rest of the digestive system the energy which ordinarily is required in the digestion of food is free to be diverted to the work of elimination. It would seem that under these circumstances all of the functions of the body are especially active in the blood-purifying processes.

You should remember, however, that even a fast will naturally be made much more effective by the general blood-purifying methods which I have given in this chapter. The measures suggested for increasing the activity of the skin will all be especially valuable if employed as adjuncts to the fast. The free drinking of water and especially the hot-water-drinking plan, together with the colon-flushing treatment, will likewise help to facilitate the cleansing and blood-purifying action of the fast.

Pure blood is the all-important factor in health. If the blood is not pure it can be made pure by the methods which I have suggested. Remember that this purity depends first upon pure food and functional strength, in order that a good quality of blood may be produced; and secondly, upon active elimination of wastes, poisons and impurities in general.

CHAPTER XVII: Hints on Bathing

I have already referred to the value of accelerating the activity of the functions of the skin. The ordinary practice of bathing is of great importance in this connection. Many diseases would be prevented if the skin were thoroughly cleansed with due regularity.

Probably a weekly soap-and-water bath is all that is absolutely essential for cleanliness if one follows a daily regimen which will maintain a condition of internal cleanliness. In fact, the cleansing of the external body is not required with such frequency if one secures sufficient muscular exercise and follows a dietetic and general regimen that will guarantee sufficient activity of all the eliminative functions; but if one neglects to employ other measures that help to maintain the purity of the blood and the activity of the skin, then more frequent baths are required to insure cleanliness. It has been my custom to recommend a hot soap-and-water bath once or twice a week, depending upon the individual requirements, and a daily cold bath. The hot bath is to be used as a cleansing agent while the cold bath is a tonic exclusively. A regimen of this sort will usually be satisfactory where one is taking a general system of exercise nearly every day which will insure a certain amount of internal functional activity. Note, however, that the cold bath, though of some value, is not necessary, when following the hot-water-drinking regimen.

There has been much controversy as to whether or not cold baths are really beneficial, since in some cases they have proved harmful. Under such circumstances the failure to secure good results may have been due to ignorance of the principles involved and to the lack of vitality essential to reaction from the shock of the cold water. A great deal depends upon the manner in which the cold bath is taken and the physical condition of the individual taking it.

A cold bath is a strong stimulant to the entire circulatory system, provided one can recuperate with a feeling of warmth immediately thereafter. If this feeling of warmth does not follow, if you feel cold, uncomfortable, nervous and trembling for some time after the bath, the shock has been too severe and is not of advantage. Under such circumstances it is better either to avoid the bath altogether or else take more exercise in order more thoroughly to warm the body before taking the bath. Usually if one is warm before bathing and if the cold bath is taken in a warm room it is easy to recuperate from it. Another good suggestion in a case of this kind is to decrease the duration of the bath. Do not stay in the water too long. In some cases what is sometimes called a hand bath may be advantageous. This bath is taken by merely wetting the hands several times in the water and applying the moist palms to all parts of the body. The familiar sponge bath, so-called, using either a sponge or a washcloth, is often advised, although the hand bath just mentioned is even easier to take.

I have also frequently recommended the use of the dry friction bath, following exercise, as a means of preparing the body for a cold bath. I have already referred to these dry friction rubbings as a means of accelerating the activity of the skin. This friction bath will, in nearly all cases, warm the skin sufficiently to enable one thoroughly to enjoy the cold water. In fact, this friction is to a cold bath what appetite is to eating. You should enjoy your meals and you should enjoy your cold bath. It is only when the cold bath is a pleasure that it is a benefit. If you dread it, if the mere thought of taking a cold bath brings a shudder, it will not be of benefit to you. You should feel sufficiently vigorous and vital really to enjoy it. A friction bath will put your skin in a condition where the cold water will "feel good." Exercise that thoroughly warms the body will naturally have the same effect.

The statement has often been made that to take a cold bath when overheated is dangerous just as it would be to drink a large amount of very cold water when overheated. It is said that one should wait until he cools off before taking the cold drink or cold plunge. To a limited extent there is wisdom in this advice, especially as it applies to getting into cold water when overheated and then remaining there until you have cooled off. Such quick cooling is certainly dangerous, just as drinking too much very cold water is dangerous. On the other hand, a short quick cold bath under such circumstances is not dangerous but highly advisable. The danger in such cases lies in remaining in the water until chilled. As a matter of fact, when one is overheated he can thoroughly enjoy the cold water. You will recuperate quickly under such conditions and you can better afford to take a cold bath when very hot than when chilled. Do not attempt cold bathing when you have "goose flesh" or when your hands and feet are cold. Under such circumstances the hand bath is preferable. It is always best when overheated to cool off gradually, and after the bath taken under such circumstances to use a sweater or bath robe or other covering to insure the desired result. When one is overheated, it is best to drink water lukewarm or hot or only moderately cool. If you drink lukewarm water when overheated you can take any quantity desired.

As previously stated, however, I would like to point out that if you are carrying out the regimen of hot-water-drinking and exercise previously referred to, a daily cold bath is not at all necessary. It might be taken with benefit if you are vigorous, but by flushing the body with a large amount of liquid according to the plan I have suggested virtually all functions of the body, including that of the skin itself, are accelerated in their activities. Under such circumstances less bathing is required, at least for the purpose of maintaining proper circulation and functional activity. Therefore the question may be left open for each individual to determine. One may take a cold bath or not, just as he may desire, while following the regimen referred to.

Many who enjoy a cold bath are inclined to stay in the water too long. In this way one may deprive himself of some of the benefits that might be derived therefrom. It is safer to limit the cold bath to a short period. The chief value lies in the reaction. If this is secured then all is well. The first effect of the cold water is to contract the tissues at the surface of the body, including the blood vessels, thus forcing the blood away from the skin. In the reaction the blood is brought back to the surface in large quantities, producing the glow that is noticed after a successful cold bath. After a short plunge or quick shower this reaction should be secured. By staying in the water too long one may overtax his vitality and become chilled. When taking a plunge simply allow the water to come in contact with all parts of the body; then immediately get out.

If the recuperative powers are defective you should not use cold water, though the hand bath as described should be satisfactory. In such cases, however, by maintaining the warmth of the feet you can recuperate quickly and easily. If you will stand with your feet in hot water while taking the hand bath, or sponge bath, or when using a hand spray in the bathtub, recuperation will be easier. When the feet are warm the circulation is more easily maintained. Following a hot bath, the hand spray can be used for the shower, applying the water quickly to all parts of the body before getting out of the tub. One should always use a cold sponge, spray, or shower, after a hot bath to close the pores. Then rub dry quickly and vigorously with a Turkish towel.

A sitz bath is recommended instead of a full tub bath, as it is a tonic of great value through its effect upon certain sympathetic nerve centers. This bath consists in immersing only the central part of the body, namely, the hips and abdomen. Special sitz tubs are manufactured, but one can use an ordinary wash tub. An ordinary bathtub will serve if filled with water about six to ten inches deep. Put the feet on the edge of the tub and lower the hips down into the water. This bath is especially valuable as a means of stimulating functional activity. The colder the water for the sitz bath the better, although if one is lacking in vitality, it should not be below 70 degrees Fahrenheit. A hot sitz bath may sometimes be suggested for inflammatory and painful conditions in the pelvic region. In inflammation of the bladder, for instance, it is valuable.

When taking hot baths for cleansing purposes the soap used is of some importance; especially so if the skin is thin or too dry. In such cases strong soaps are injurious, although their effect may be overcome to some extent by rubbing the body after the bath with a very little bit of olive oil. I would suggest, however, the use of a pure vegetable oil soap, such as castile, which is one of the best examples of a vegetable soap. This soap may be suggested in all cases, but it is particularly important when the skin is thin or dry. Very frequently dryness of skin is noticed in those of very light complexion. In the preceding chapter on Blood Purification I referred to a hot bath for the purpose of rapidly eliminating poisons and wastes in the body. An ordinary warm bath for cleansing purposes need not be taken at such a high temperature. In other words a soap-and-water bath will be perfectly satisfactory at a temperature of 103 to 105 degrees F. and need not occupy more than a very few minutes, whereas the hot bath referred to for the special purpose of blood purification may be of longer duration and of a much higher temperature, running up to 110 or 115 degrees Fahrenheit.

There is another type of warm bath, however, which is of special value in many cases. This is what I have sometimes termed a neutral bath, inasmuch as it is neither hot nor cold. This is a bath at about the temperature of the body, that is to say, 95 to 98 degrees Fahrenheit. One should use a bath thermometer to be sure of the right temperature. This neutral bath has a sedative or quieting effect upon the nerves through its effect upon the innumerable nerve endings in the skin. It is neither hot nor cold, neither stimulating nor weakening, and one could remain in such a bath for hours without harm. It has a quieting effect upon the nerves and reference has been made to it in the chapter on Sleep as a means of overcoming excitement or nervousness. In attacks of mania it is especially valuable, and is now extensively used in all insane asylums because of its wonderful effect in quieting the nerves. This bath at 98 degrees is also especially commended in the case of severe burns covering a large surface. It is about the only way in which a person suffering from such an extensive burn can be made comfortable. It is also one of the most perfect forms of treatment in a case of that kind. The serious character of the burn depends not so much upon the severity as upon the extent of the surface involved. Therefore, one who has been seriously burned could remain immersed in a bath at 98 degrees F. for many days continuously, or until the skin has had a chance to heal. Immersion in water is a natural condition, for there was a time away back when all the animal life of the earth was found in the water. It was only through special variation in the character of evolution that certain forms of life finally became adapted to a life outside of the water. Therefore, immersion in water, except for the head, is not entirely an unnatural condition.

CHAPTER XVIII: Some Facts About Clothing

The statement is often heard that a man is made or marred by the clothes he wears. This is frequently said with a view to emphasizing the importance of being presentably appareled, but it has a meaning beyond this. To a certain extent we are really made, or we may more properly say marred, by the clothes we wear. Civilized costumes have become what they are through the dictation of the creators of style, the clothing manufacturers. Every year the styles change through the commands of those whose profits are increased by this continual variation in the fashions. It is said that a woman would rather be out of the world than out of style. Therefore, each year she discards her old-style costumes and buys the latest modes.

We have to recognize, however, that clothing is a necessary evil at this period of human progress, so-called. There was a time when clothing was worn entirely as a matter of protection or as a means of adding warmth to the body. There was no thought given to the necessity for covering the body, for every part of the human anatomy was as commonplace as nose, fingers and toes. But now clothing is commanded as a means of hiding our bodily contour. Prudery has come in and branded the human anatomy as indecent and consequently it must be covered.

Now in considering what we should wear we are compelled to adhere, at least to a reasonable extent, to what we call style, but beyond this our first thought must be for bodily comfort. And in speaking of comfort we mean not only the warmth essential to this but also the ability to
use every part of our bodily structure with as little restraint as possible. If we could wear a costume which would permit us to feel just as free and untrammeled in our movements as we do when without clothing such a form of dress would be ideal. Our movements should not be restricted by our clothing any more than is absolutely unavoidable. The ordinary skirt, supposed to be a necessary part of feminine apparel, Is in its nature an evil of first importance. Every step taken by a woman wearing such a garment is hampered; she is continuously handicapped

by her skirt. If a man were compelled to walk through tall, heavy grass all his life he would get some idea of the extent to which the feminine skirt interferes with the freedom of woman.

Numerous other defects of our costumes interfere with bodily freedom. Take our tight and ungainly shoes. Here is an abominable instance of our slavery to style. In most instances the foot is made to fit the shoe, and the suffering that is endured by many so-called stylish people for the purpose of making the foot fit the shoe would be difficult to describe. A shoe should fit the foot. The more nearly you approximate the same freedom when walking in a shoe as you do when barefooted the more perfect the shoe. The toes should not be squeezed out of shape. The great toe should follow the straight line of the inside of the foot instead of being bent over to the position normally occupied by the middle toe. All the toes should be allowed to spread out in the shoe, at least to a reasonable extent. Furthermore, a shoe that really fits should feel comfortable the first time it is put on. There should be no necessity for "breaking in" a shoe.

The artificial heel added to the ordinary shoe is another curious freak of fashion. If the Almighty in perfecting the human foot had found a high heel necessary it would have been provided. The artificial heel, especially the very high heel commonly used on shoes worn by women, is an insult to Nature, to the Creator. Some day, when we are really civilized, high heels will be unknown. I am convinced that the Omnipotent Creator knew his business thoroughly when he created the human foot, that the sole of the human foot, heel included, was made for locomotion, and that it is impossible for human ingenuity to improve upon the foot. In other words, if you can secure footwear that will enable you to walk with the same freedom that you can enjoy when barefooted, you will then have attained perfection in foot covering. Sandals and moccasins allow the feet the same freedom as one enjoys when barefooted. The sole of these forms of footwear has the same freedom in gripping the ground and adapting itself to the requirements of every step as the bare foot, and it is a curious and yet significant fact that whereas more or less foot trouble is the rule rather than the exception among civilized peoples, yet those races who wear moccasins or sandals, or go barefooted, never have flatfoot, broken arches, bunions or other defects of this type.

Passing to the other extreme of the body, our tight hats should be condemned. Hats should be as light as possible and should not be so tight as to interfere with the circulation of the scalp. Many bald headed men owe their loss of hair to tight hats. The stiff collars worn everywhere at the present time mar the natural contour of the neck, make an erect position more difficult, and are one cause of the round shoulders that are so common everywhere to-day. The suspenders worn by men have also an influence of this sort. They are inclined to pull the shoulders forward and make it more difficult to maintain an erect position. The flat-chested man will not feel his suspenders, but the man with a full round chest, properly carried, is under continuous pressure from his suspenders.

If I were to select an ideal costume for men I am inclined to think that I would go back to the Roman toga, to the flowing drapery of the Greeks, or to the Scottish kilt. The kilt is undoubtedly better suited than the robe to the colder weather of Northern Europe and America. These costumes not only allow a reasonable amount of freedom for all bodily movements, encouraging rather than discouraging the correct position of the body, but they also allow free circulation of air to the central portions of the body. As a hygienic feature this is of tremendous value. The air coming in contact with the skin is of value at all times, but it is especially required in these important parts of the bodily organism. Many weaknesses are brought about through the unhealthful covering and restriction of these parts. Trousers are not by any means an ideal garment. To be sure, they are a vast improvement over the long skirt, but they are not by any means equal in healthfulness to the costume of the Scottish Highlanders.

In feminine apparel corsets are perhaps productive of more injury than any other part of the costume. The injury wrought by tight lacing is now everywhere understood, and in recent years large waists have become stylish. This tendency of the times will ultimately mean the elimination of the corset.

When fully clothed we should have the same freedom of movement as when unclothed. The most perfect costume is our "birthday clothing," the clothing with which we came into the world, the human skin. To be sure, in cold climates bodily covering is necessary for warmth a part of the year, though in warm climates, or warm seasons, the more nearly we avoid restrictive apparel, the more happy and more healthy we are. The ideal costume in warm weather, therefore, would be no costume, but conventions demand that we cover our nakedness, and this command should be followed in a manner that will restrain our movements as little as possible.

The question of color is an important factor in clothing. This is especially true in summer when exposure to the sun makes it especially necessary to consider our comfort. All dark-colored clothing absorbs the heat and the sun becomes very oppressive to the wearer. Then, too, black and dark-colored coverings shut out the light, another objectionable feature. In my reference to sun baths in the preceding chapter on Blood Purification I placed special emphasis upon the value of light as a vitalizing and stimulating factor in life and health. Ordinarily we not only smother our skins so far as the air is concerned, but we also shut out the light, hiding our bodies in a cellar, so to speak. Our bodies need light as well as air and for this reason dark colored clothing cannot be recommended. For warmth when in the sunshine during the winter, black is very effective. When out of the sunshine black is cooler in winter than light-colored fabrics because it quickly radiates the body heat. It is well known that a black stove radiates the heat much faster than a nickel-plated or brightly polished stove.

White or light-colored garments are advised in summer, both because they are cooler and because they permit the light to reach the skin. The Arabs, Bedouins and others who live in unforested countries where they are much exposed to the tropical sun use turbans and flowing robes of white as a means of keeping cool. Pure white is often unserviceable, because it quickly becomes soiled, and therefore gray and tan- colored garments are recommended.

It is easily possible to absorb too much sunshine, especially in the lower latitudes. The various races of the earth enjoy a degree of pigmentation of the skin corresponding to the intensity of the sunlight in the latitude to which they have become accustomed through the course of evolution. Equatorial races are black, far-northern races are blonde with very fair skin, and those occupying mean latitudes are either brown or olive-hued. Brunettes or fairly dark-complexioned white men can stand more sunshine than the blue-eyed, fair-skinned types of Scotland, Norway and Sweden. Where the latter are exposed to intensely strong sunshine in latitudes further south than their natural home, and especially when visiting the tropics, where the sun's rays are nearly vertical, some special protection from the excessive light is necessary. Then the upper or outer clothing should be white or light-colored, but an undergarment of some opaque or dark-colored material should be used to shut out the light. In the case of tropical animals Nature provides a light-colored or tawny growth of hair, with an underlying black or heavily pigmented skin. The white man when in the tropics or when subject to the chemical rays of the sun in midsummer would do well to follow Nature's example, wearing light clothing outside with black- or orange-colored or other opaque underwear. The hat should be white or tan or light-colored on top, but with a dark-colored lining extending under the brim. Blonde types spending the summer in a latitude like that of Texas or Mexico would do well to consider these suggestions. Sunlight is essential to life. Sun baths are invaluable and ordinarily our clothing should be such as to permit the light to reach the skin. But when the sun's rays are nearly vertical fair-skinned persons may easily protect themselves and maintain comfort by following this suggestion.

As a general thing, during both winter and summer, one should wear no more clothing than necessary, and that should be of a type to permit easy access of air to the skin. For this reason the character of one's underwear is important. Wool is undoubtedly warmer and more or less suitable for exceptionally cold weather; yet for most purposes linen is to be preferred because of its more porous character. Linen permits of free circulation of the air, and when the underwear is woven with an open mesh it is especially satisfactory. Next to linen cotton is to be preferred, being likewise porous. The question of underwear is one to be determined largely by individual taste and requirements, but always it should be understood that one should wear underwear as light as is consistent with warmth and as porous as possible. This principle should also apply in the matter of shoes. Air-tight foot coverings are highly detrimental as well as uncomfortable. Leather in its natural state is porous and therefore a healthful foot covering. Patent-leather shoes, however, have been made air-tight by a special process, and are very hot, uncomfortable and unsanitary. The sole of the shoe should consist of nothing but plain leather. So-called waterproofing processes, making the shoe air-tight as well as waterproof, should be avoided. Patented, waterproof soles are highly objectionable. If you can have your shoes made to order see to it that the sole consists of nothing but leather-indeed a single layer of good sole leather is most satisfactory. Although such shoes will absorb water they will dry readily, and the disadvantage of wet feet on occasions is more than offset by the benefits gained from a porous foot covering the rest of the time. Anyway, wet feet are unimportant if the feet are warm.

A word about winter clothing. Heavy underclothing is entirely unsuited to the temperatures maintained inside our houses during the winter. We usually have a summer temperature indoors in winter and should wear summer clothing. It is true that we require warmer clothing out-of-doors in winter, but this should be used only when out-of-doors; we should not wear heavy, warm garments both indoors and out. Therefore, while the farmer who spends the day in the open would probably need heavy warm underwear, the city man should dress approximately the same as in summer when indoors, and add the garments necessary for additional warmth when going out. Sweaters, gaiters and overcoats should be depended on when going out-of-doors instead of heavy undergarments.

Clothing, as I have said, is a necessary evil. So far as possible it should not hamper our movements and should not deprive our bodies of light and air. Since it is necessary to wear clothing, I would strongly emphasize the importance of taking air baths at frequent intervals. When spending the evening in the privacy of your own room, studying or writing letters, you have a good opportunity to enjoy an air bath during the entire evening. And furthermore, when at home you should lay aside your coat and use no more bodily covering than is necessary. If you cannot take sun baths at a special hour each day, then I would advise that when taking your walk out-of-doors in the sunshine you wear clothing of such a character as to admit the rays of the sun, thus enabling you to enjoy a sun bath during your walk. A special suit of clothes, made of natural-colored linen, with a thin light shirt, light-colored socks and no underwear, would answer all purposes admirably.

CHAPTER XIX: Suggestions About Sleep

Sleep is one of the first essentials in maintaining or in building vitality. There are differences of opinion as to how much sleep may be necessary to health, but that sufficient sleep is required if one wishes to maintain the maximum of energy no one can question.

Sleep is far more necessary than food. One can fast for many days, or many weeks if necessary, and without any special disadvantage if he is well nourished before beginning the fast and has a satisfactory food supply after ifs conclusion, but no one can "fast" from sleep for more than a few days at a time without experiencing ill effects. One can scarcely endure an entire week of absolute sleeplessness. It has been found that dogs kept awake even though sufficiently fed, suffer more than when deprived of food and permitted to sleep. When kept awake continuously they die in four or five days. Man can endure the strain a little longer than the dogs, but five or six days usually marks the limit of human life under such conditions. In early English history condemned criminals were put to death by being deprived of sleep, and the same method has been employed in China. Enforced sleeplessness, in fact, has been used as a form of torture by the Chinese, being more feared than any other. The men subjected to this frightful ordeal always die raving maniacs.

These facts illustrate only too well the imperative necessity for sleep. Unfortunately "late hours" prevail, especially in large cities. Manifestly, if complete lack of sleep is fatal, late hours and partial lack of sleep is at least devitalizing and detrimental to health. The late hours kept by large numbers of people in civilized countries undoubtedly contribute very largely to neurasthenia and allied diseases. Improvements in artificial lights have contributed largely toward the increase of the evil of late hours, injurious not only through the loss of sleep entailed, but also because of the eye-strain incidental to strong artificial lights and the drain on the nervous system. If civilized man would follow the example of primitive man and of many of the birds and animals in retiring to bed with the coming of darkness and arising with the appearance of daylight, this one change would revolutionize the health of the whole human race. How much sleep do we need? This is a question that cannot be answered arbitrarily as applying in all cases. Individuals differ. Without doubt, some require more sleep than others.

Thomas A. Edison, who is an extraordinary man, not only in respect to his vitality but in every other characteristic as well, has frequently been quoted as saying that most men and women sleep too much. Mr. Edison himself claims to maintain the best of health with from three to five hours' sleep out of every twenty-four. We have heard of other cases too, of men and women with exceptional vitality, who have seemed to thrive on four or five hours' sleep. It is possible that this small allowance of sleep may be sufficient in such cases, but if so, it is undoubtedly due to the exceptionally powerful organism which these particular persons have inherited.

No definite rule can be laid down as to the amount of sleep required by different individuals, for those possessing the greatest amount of vitality and the strongest organisms will require less sleep than those of limited vitality and weak functional powers. Those possessing a strong functional system and great vitality are able to build up energy during sleep and recuperate from the exertions of the preceding day more rapidly than can those less favored in this respect. In other words, a very strong man can be quickly rested. His system can more rapidly than that of a weak man repair the wear and tear of his daily work. The man or woman with limited strength and a less vigorous functional system would require a longer time in which to recuperate. Therefore, what would hold good in the case of such an extraordinary man as Mr. Edison cannot be depended upon in the case of the average man or woman, and certainly will not meet the needs of those who are debilitated and striving to build vitality.

Generally speaking, therefore, I maintain that most people at the present day sleep too little rather than too much. I would not stipulate any special number of hours for sleeping but I would advise everyone to secure as much sleep as he requires. It has often been said that if you sleep too much you will be stupid as a result. Such results are usually

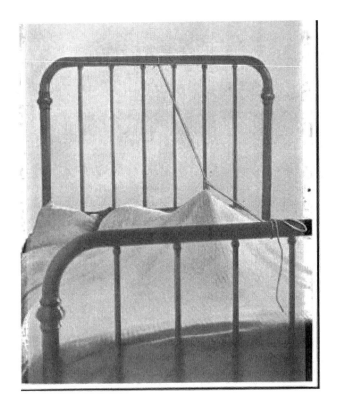

Illustrating an idea for removing the weight of the coverings from the body while sleeping. A heavy cord is fastened to the foot and head of the bed and the covers are hung from the cord by the aid of a very large safety pin. This idea will enable one to sleep throughout the entire night in what might be termed an air bath.

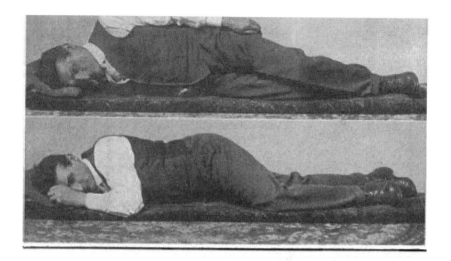

Showing an ideal position for sleeping. In order to assume this position
properly, lie on the side with the wrist under the small part of the waist,
the hand just showing as is illustrated in the upper picture. Now roll
over until the body is in the position shown in the lower picture, weight
of the upper body resting on elbows and chest. In this position it will be
noted that the abdomen has perfect freedom to fully expand

brought about by sleeping in unsatisfactory environment, particularly in stuffy rooms in which the air is vitiated and really unfit to breathe. I cannot imagine one feeling stupid as a result of oversleeping when sleeping out-of-doors, or when the supply of air is absolutely fresh.

Excessive heat would probably be conducive to restlessness, but this is purely a detail which I shall take up later. Under natural and healthful conditions one will rarely sleep too much. If you sleep until you wake up naturally there is little danger of your sleeping too much. Without doubt most people need from seven to eight hours' sleep; some of them need more, particularly women and children, who in many cases require from nine to ten hours' sleep or even more. These are general statements. Individual exceptions will be many, but, as I have said, it will be found that those who need less sleep are men and women of extraordinary vitality.

The quality of sleep is really more important than the duration of sleep. It is quality or depth of sleep that is really what counts, and to secure this it is necessary that certain healthful conditions be observed. The first of these is a normal condition of physical or muscular fatigue. This is easily distinguished from nervous fatigue or exhaustion in which the entire system is more or less upset. Abnormal states of this sort arise from excitement, excessive mental work, or other conditions involving severe nerve strain. This nervous fatigue is not usually conducive to sleep, but a tired condition of the muscles of the body generally, as a result of natural physical activity, is always favorable to sleep. Many who complain of insomnia, therefore, would often be able to remedy their trouble by the simple expedient of a long walk, covering sufficient distance to bring about the physical fatigue which makes sleep possible. Conditions of air, temperature and bed covering are also important factors in connection with the quality of sleep.

If you are a sound sleeper it may be possible for you to secure more benefit from three to four hours' sleep than a shallow sleeper may secure in eight hours of a lighter degree of sleep. This extreme depth of sleep means complete rest for the brain, absolute loss of consciousness, and, to a certain extent, loss of sensibility in respect to our senses. In the lighter degree of sleep certain parts of the brain may be at rest, while others are more or less active. Dreaming represents a state of partial consciousness rather than a condition of complete rest, inasmuch as various parts of the brain are active. One may thus be conscious of his dreams. There is no doubt, however, that in other cases various parts of the brain may be active though we may not be conscious of their activity. We have all heard of instances where mathematical problems appear to have been worked out during sleep, and we have heard of musical compositions and poems being produced during sleep. All these phenomena represent a condition in which one is partly asleep and partly awake; in other words, some parts of the brain are active and others are asleep. In extreme depth of sleep when all the mental faculties are at rest, the energies are relaxed, and the activities of the body are at a low ebb; it is such sound sleep that makes for rapid recuperation. The deepest sleep generally occurs within the first few hours after falling to sleep, and it gradually becomes lighter and lighter in degree until consciousness is reached. Dreams, therefore, represent partial consciousness and usually appear in the earlier hours of the morning. When one states that he dreams all night he is invariably mistaken. One may seem to live over periods of days and even years in a dream, the actual duration of which may be measured in minutes. The chances are that the dreamer enjoyed a sound sleep before his dreaming commenced.

Although I have said that depth of sleep is more important than the duration of sleep, yet it is true that when one sleeps very soundly he usually sleeps longer. In other words, when one reaches great depth of sleep the transition to the period of wakefulness is only gradual, and it requires a longer time to complete the sleep and wake up than it would if one did not sleep so deeply, or, as we would say, so soundly. It will be found that healthy children, who unquestionably sleep very soundly, also sleep for many hours at a time. They may have dreams but these occur in the later hours of sleep, as every mother has observed. The man or woman well advanced in years who can secure the same depth of sleep that a vigorous child enjoys will undoubtedly spend the bigger part of the night in sleep and will acquire exceptional vitality as a result.

Bodily rest, even without sleep, is undoubtedly of great value for purposes of recuperation. To a certain extent such rest, especially if associated with a state of very complete relaxation of the muscles, will make it possible to take less sleep without serious devitalizing results. The man or woman who suffers from insomnia should learn that he can recuperate to a considerable extent through simple physical relaxation without the unconsciousness of sleep. Undoubtedly the physical inactivity common among civilized races has much to do with their ability to keep late hours. But of course this involves more or less nerve strain. The brain does not get sufficient rest, and the loss of sleep involves such an expenditure of energy through the brain as to constitute a serious drain upon the nervous system. Even though rest for the body during consciousness is of certain value, it cannot go very far in taking the place of true sleep. To the higher centers of the brain and nervous system an opportunity must be given for the complete relaxation that comes only with the entire loss of consciousness.

As I have already said, those who are lacking in vitality and who are trying to build strength need more sleep than those who are already strong. Especially those who find it difficult to sleep need additional nervous strength and should carefully observes rules that will promote sleep. One will often hear sufferers from insomnia complain that they never sleep! They are convinced that night after night and week after week passes without their being able to close their eyes in slumber. They are deluded in every case, because they could not maintain life for more than five or six days if this were true. The fact is that they drop off to sleep and then awaken without being conscious that they have been asleep. At the same time, in all such conditions, it is necessary to improve the quality of sleep so that it will be truly refreshing. I have already referred to the influence of good healthy muscular fatigue as a means of enabling one to sleep.

Walking and out-of-door life will in almost every case make the nervous man or woman sleep like a child. One should not be too fatigued, but sufficiently so to thoroughly enjoy the sensation of lying down. One cannot truly enjoy sleep except when he has reached this condition of bodily fatigue. To induce this, I would recommend a walk in the evening before going to bed, covering several miles. Although walking for health should ordinarily be brisk enough to stimulate breathing and arouse an active circulation, thus strengthening the internal organs, for the purpose of promoting drowsiness the last mile or two of the evening walk should preferably be very slow. Fast movements are stimulating to mind and nerves. Slow movements have a sedative effect. By walking very slowly as if one were tired the desired effect of fatigue is more satisfactorily secured. One imagines the need of rest under such conditions.

The quality of the air is another important factor, though I need not dwell upon that here. The air you breathe during sleep should be especially fresh and pure, particularly so because of the more shallow character of the breathing. If you are in a room, all the windows should be open as wide as possible. If you have a covered balcony or porch, or if you can avail yourself of a flat roof, it is always advisable to sleep out-of-doors. The increased vitality will more than repay you for your trouble. There is something about out-of-door sleeping that vitalizes, energizes, and refreshes one to an unusual extent.

Circulation is another important factor in sound sleep, especially for nervous persons. Many of those who complain of an inability to sleep suffer more or less from congestion of blood in the brain; also they complain of cold feet or cold hands and feet. In such instances, warm feet will often bring a solution of the problem. In some instances drinking a half cup of hot milk or hot water before going to bed will draw the blood from the brain and enable one to sleep. A hot foot bath before going to bed will do the same thing, or one may use a hot-water bag or hot flatiron wrapped up in flannels, or even a hot brick treated in the same way, to keep the feet warm when in bed. In extreme cases it might be advisable to apply cold packs to the head while applying heat to the feet or when taking the hot foot bath.

Another measure of special value for nervous persons is a bath at the temperature of the body, to be taken for a half-hour before going to sleep. In cases of extreme excitement, anger or nervousness this bath is invaluable. Fill the tub with water at 96 degrees Fahrenheit or 98 degrees Fahrenheit. You can remain in this bath for several hours without harm, for it is neither weakening nor stimulating. It has a soothing effect upon the nerves and is even valuable in preventing attacks of hysteria or other nervous difficulties. This particular bath is so effective in hospitals for the insane that it has frequently obviated the use of padded cells and straight jackets. It is just as effective for the nervous person who wishes to overcome the excitement that is preventing sleep. A half-hour bath should be sufficient for ordinary purposes. Another remedy of great value for soothing the nerves is the air bath. I have referred to this in another part of this volume, but it is extremely valuable for quieting the nerves in cases of insomnia. If the room is comfortably warm, an air bath can be advantageously taken for half an hour before going to bed.

One of the most valuable remedies for those suffering from sleeplessness is to lie in an air bath during the entire night. This idea can be carried out very easily by raising the bed covering in such a way as to remove its weight from the body, thus providing what we might call a chamber of air in which to sleep. With the aid of a large safety-pin or a horse-blanket safety-pin, the bed clothing may be kept thus suspended. The safety-pin is pinned through all the coverings in the center of the bed and then by means of a string passing through the safety-pin and running from the to of the head of the bed to the top of the foot of the bed the bed covering can easily be raised to the desired height. The appearance of the bed is then somewhat like that of a small tent. One may not feel warm immediately after entering, if the weather is cold, but if the covering is thick enough and the air is entirely excluded, a perfect air bath, warm and comfortable, can be enjoyed during the entire night. The head, of course, will keep its usual position outside of the covers. No underclothing or night clothing should be worn when attempting to carry out this idea.

The problems associated with covering are of considerable importance. Many people are unable to sleep because of cold feet and many are overheated by an excess of covering. It should not be necessary to bury one's self underneath a heavy load of covers in order to keep the feet warm. Use as little covering as possible and still maintain the bodily warmth. Eider-down bed covers are very valuable because of their light weight and great warmth-retaining qualities. Overheating during sleep produces restlessness and robs one of the sense of refreshment on awakening. The question of cold feet I have already dealt with. The difficulty, in most cases, is one of defective circulation before going to bed. If one will be sure that his feet are warm and his circulation good before retiring to bed he will invariably have no trouble of this kind, even during winter time. I do not mean that one should be chilled by insufficient bedding, but I certainly would advise as little covering as is compatible with a comfortable degree of warmth.

The feather beds, much used in Europe, are undesirable, as they are unsanitary and are too warm for nearly all seasons of the year. It is always best to sleep between clean linen sheets. For purposes of warmth, however, bear in mind that cotton is of very little value, whereas animal-product covers such as wool and down, or feathers, are exceptionally warm. Cotton comforters in cold weather are very heavy, but cold, whereas woolen blankets, wool-filled comforters or down-filled comforters are warm, but light. "A warmth without weight" should be the chief consideration in cold weather. And in using woolen coverings you can get sufficient warmth without much weight and with the very least quantity of covering. In summer use only a single woolen blanket or a light cotton coverlet over the sheet. When the nights are hot and sultry it would be well to use no covering of any kind.

For warmth in winter special attention should be given to warm fabrics underneath the lower sheet as well as the coverings. One may become chilled from underneath if lying upon a thin mattress or an uncovered mattress. A wool-filled comforter, or double woolen blanket, placed over the mattress and under the sheet will contribute greatly to one's warmth. If the mattress is of proper thickness one can be comfortable with less covering and therefore less weight. However, I would suggest as a better plan the one that I have presented of sleeping in a virtual air bath the whole night through.

The use of a pillow is necessary in nearly all cases. When one is sleeping on his back a pillow is certainly an objectionable feature. It tips the head forward and is conducive to round shoulders. A pillow is of value when sleeping on the side or in the partial face-downward position, as indicated in the illustration.

The accompanying illustration shows a special position that I can recommend for securing restful sleep and for insuring deeper respiration. In this position you sleep with the body tipped forward partly upon the chest, and on the forearm, with one elbow just back of the body and hand under the waist. The knee of the upper leg will be drawn up somewhat. While this is a very comfortable position its chief advantage lies in the effect upon the respiration. It will be noted that in this position the organs lying below the diaphragm are placed in a suspended position, so to speak. The stomach and other organs by their own weight pull downward from the diaphragm, thus naturally allowing more space in the lungs, and particularly in the lower part of the lungs. Through the simple effect of gravitation, therefore, this position allows one to breathe a larger amount of air through the entire night. One may turn from one side to the other in order to change the position, as it will be equally comfortable on right or left sides. In cases where there is weakness of the heart the left-side position can not be recommended if discomfort of any sort is noticed.

One often hears a reference to beauty sleep and is often asked: "Is it really true that an hour of sleep before midnight is equal to two hours after midnight?" There are many writers who claim that the time when you sleep matters but little if you secure a sufficient amount of sleep. It is doubtful, however, if this view is absolutely correct. I am inclined to lean towards the old-fashioned view as to the good effect of early retiring on beauty development that is based on health building.

In one sense, it is reasonable to conclude that an hour of sleep before midnight is worth more than an hour thereafter. I am satisfied that there is greater exhaustion of the body from late than from normal hours, and it is difficult to get the full benefit from sleep when going to bed after midnight. At least the nerve strain of artificial light tends to produce a certain degree of vital depletion that one would not

experience if his waking hours included only the daylight.
Then again, there is probably some mysterious influence that we do
not fully comprehend which makes sleep at night more restful than
sleep during the daylight. Those who go to bed at midnight or
thereafter use several hours of daylight in the early morning for
sleeping. I realize that there are nocturnal animals and that the human
race has developed nocturnal habits to a certain extent, but the human
race and the animal life of the world generally have followed the habit
through the ages of sleeping at night. Without doubt a revolutionary
change in this habit has more or less effect upon the restful character of
our sleep. Perhaps the mere question of light has much to do with it.
Daylight is stimulating. Light has a chemical action and tends
to stimulate animal metabolism. Darkness, or the lack of light, tends
to a restful condition. Without doubt this question of light has much to
do with the supposed benefits of sleep before midnight. The old saying
that "early to bed and early to rise makes a man healthy, wealthy and
wise" may not hold true in the matter of wisdom and wealth in all
cases, but there is no doubt it has much to do with the development of
health and vitality.

CHAPTER XX:
Mind - The Master-Force for Health or Disease

We hear of many miraculous achievements in the building of health and the cure of disease through mental influence. The mind is unquestionably a master-force. I will not go so far as to say it is limitless, for certainly a hungry man cannot imagine he is eating a dinner and secure the same benefits that he would from the meal itself. Nor can a man who is passing away into the other world, through a definite vital defect, bring back life through mental force.

But we should remember that many diseases are to a great extent imaginary. And some of those not actually imaginary may at least be brought about through fears that are the results of abnormal delusions. And where such diseases are combated by mental forces of the right sort, a cure can be effected in many instances. In numerous cases, also, it is well to remember that the mental state is the actual cause of disease. You become blue, hopeless and to a certain extent helpless. You see nothing in the future. Life is dull. Ambition, enthusiasm, have all disappeared. It would not be at all difficult for this state of mind to bring about disease in some form.

Health, strength, vitality of the right sort, should radiate all the elements and forces associated with life's most valuable possessions. Happiness and health are close friends. It is very difficult to be gloomy and miserable if you are healthy. It is perhaps even more difficult to be healthy if you are gloomy and mentally ugly.

Therefore it is a wise precaution to cultivate a hopeful spirit. If the day is gloomy, if the sun is obscured by clouds, then develop the sunshine in your own spirit. Try to radiate good cheer. By seeking to cheer up others you will cheer yourself up, for always when we help others, we inevitably help ourselves, though this should not be our main purpose in the action. When we try to build up the characters, improve the morals and add to the mental and physical stability of others our efforts develop our own powers. Therefore, the best way to help yourself is to help others.

BERNARR MACFADDEN

We have a remarkable exemplification of the value of mental influence in what is known as Christian Science. Even the most prejudiced enemy of this cult will admit that many remarkable cures have been accomplished through the principles it advocates. These cures alone indicate clearly that the mind is a dominating force that works for good or for evil. They prove that your thoughts are building up or tearing down your vital forces; that to a certain extent "Thoughts are things," that good thoughts are a real tangible influence for developing mental or physical force, and-that bad thoughts have an opposite influence. It is well for each one of us to determine clearly whether the thoughts that fill our minds each day are constructive or destructive in nature.

Your thoughts can actually destroy you. They can kill you as unerringly as a bullet fired from a rifle. Keep this fact very definitely before you, and try to make your thoughts each day the means of adding to your life forces. There are many emotions that are harbored on occasions, which are devitalizing and destructive.

We are all, to a certain extent, slaves of habit, whether good or bad. For instance, there is the worrying habit, for worry is really a habit. Therefore, it is a splendid plan to become slaves of good habits. One who has acquired the chronic habit of worrying needs a mental antiseptic. Worry never benefited anyone; it has brought thousands to an untimely grave. To give prolonged and grave thought to a problem that may come into your life, with the view of forming an intelligent conclusion, should not be called worry, but anxiety. There is a very great difference between worry and concentrated study of a vexing problem. The characteristic of worry is a tendency to brood anxiously over fancied troubles. The typical worrying mind will take mere trifles and magnify them until they become monumental difficulties. Many acquire the habit of going over and over again, and still again, the various unpleasant experiences which they have passed through during life. This inclination is baneful in its influence, To such persons I would say, eliminate the past. Try the forgetting habit, cultivate health and along with it good cheer. Make your mind a blank so far as the past is concerned, and fill it with uplifting thoughts for the present and the future. Worry is a mental poison, the toxic element produced in the mind by retention of waste matter, thoughts of the dead past that should have been eliminated with the passing of out-worn periods of existence.

Self-pity is another evil. It is closely allied to worry. There are many who cultivate a mental attitude of this sort because of the sorrows through which they have passed. Such individuals find their chief delight in portraying, in vivid details, the terrific sufferings which they have had to endure. No one has suffered quite so much as they have. They harrow their friends by going over frequently and persistently the long, gruesome details of their "awful" past. This habit is destructive to an extreme degree. Why harbor past experiences that only bring sorrows to mind? Why add to the bitterness of your daily life by dragging up the lamentable past? Why pass along to your friends and acquaintances pain, sorrow and gloom? Each human entity is a radiating power. You have the capacity of passing around pain or happiness. As a rule, when you ask a friend to "have something with you" your offer is supposed to bring good cheer. You surely would not ask a friend to have pain with you, or share with you the gall of bitter, experiences through which you have lived. Therefore, if you are the victim of self-pity and if your own past sufferings discolor your every pleasant thought, at least do not taint the minds of your friends. At least keep your direful broodings to yourself if you are determined to retain them. It is, however, far wiser and manlier to avoid such thoughts, in which case your memory of these torturing experiences will gradually fade away. Live in the future and forget the past. The man or woman who lives in the future, and for the future, will invariably be optimistic and cheerful. It is a good habit to cultivate.

Then there is a mental poison called anger. Avoid it as you would a venomous snake. It has indeed been said by scientists that the venom of the snake is developed through anger, induced by impure circulation, for in reptiles the pure arterial blood mixes in the imperfectly formed heart with the impure venous blood. Scientists have also stated that anger produces a poison in the perspiration that emanates from the human body. This may or may not be true, but there is no question, however, about anger being a mental poison. It represents a tremendous waste of nervous energy. To be sure, there may be occasions when anger is justified, when it is actually desirable, but such occasions are rare. Learn to master such emotions. Get control of your feelings and mental states. Avoid useless anger definitely and finally. It usually indicates a lack of mental control, and should be recognized as a destructive force to be carefully avoided.

Hate is, to a certain extent, synonymous with anger. One may call it anger in a chronic form. Hate and the personal enmities associated with it develop emotions and characteristics that unquestionably have a destructive influence. Why hate anybody? Why waste your nervous energies by trying to "get even" with a fancied enemy? A tremendous amount of human energy is wasted in this manner. You may be impressed with the idea that someone has wronged you. You lie awake at night forming plans for "getting even." Every mental effort spent in this direction is not only destructive to body, mind and character, but it represents a waste of nervous energy. One's life should be so filled with useful activities that no time will be left for a waste of this sort. Show me a man who spends his time and efforts trying to "get even" with his supposed enemies, and I will show you a shining example of failure. No man can succeed who wastes his nervous forces in this manner.

Then there is the poison of avarice. Financial gain seems to be the one end and aim of many ambitious men. They struggle day after day and year after year in the whirlpool of perverted enthusiasm, looking continuously for wealth and still more wealth. But there is something more in life than money. Health, for instance, is worth a thousand times, and self-respect should be rated a million times, more than money. Do not allow a struggle of this sort to enslave you. Do not allow pursuits of any sort to interfere with the development and maintenance of those powers that indicate superior manhood and womanhood. It is also well to avoid the complaining and critical spirit. You will find frequent references in the Good Book to what might be termed the thankful spirit. It commands us to be thankful for what we have received. And whether or not the tenets of theology appeal to you, the thought presented is of the greatest value. If you can be thrilled each day with gladness because of the remembrance of pleasures that you have enjoyed the previous day the mental influence will be invaluable. Being thankful for what you have received does not necessarily indicate that you should not strive for more and better things. Dissatisfaction or discontent is not always necessary to spur one on to added powers and responsibilities. Avoid the complaining spirit, which will add gloom and despair to your life, no matter what may be your environment. Be thankful for the favors and opportunities that may have come to you, be they large or small, and your mental attitude in this respect will represent a potent health-building influence.

Envy is another evil it will be well to avoid, largely because it is inspired by selfish attributes. Do not envy others the joy of possessions that may be theirs. Happiness, after all, is worth but little if it comes unearned. Life's greatest pleasures are secured only through intelligent and diligent efforts. They come as the results of hard work. A man who inherits great wealth secures little or no benefit from it. It adds but little to his pleasure in life, for the greatest possible happiness comes from the pursuit rather than the attainment of an object. More happiness comes from the pursuit of wealth or pleasure than from its actual attainment. Let the attainment of truth be your aim. Truth is magnificent. It is tremendously weighted with power. Whatever your ambitions or hopes in life may be, seek for the truth. In some cases the road that leads to this goal may be devious and hard to follow. Dangers of all sorts may beset you, as you struggle along the rugged pathway that leads to truth, but the rewards will amply repay you for every effort.

Don't be a leaner. Try to stand alone. Be yourself. Bring out your own personal characteristics, do not be a stereotype, a parrot, a copy. Let others live their own lives, but you see to it that you live yours. Many of our public schools are turning out factory-made human beings; each pupil, as far as possible, a duplicate of every other. They are educational brick factories tuning out their products stamped exactly alike. Individuality is crushed out. Now the child is not so much like clay to be molded into any form, as it is like a precious crystal, that must be shaped with regard to its original nature. Each human soul is an uncut diamond. It often has within it capacities and powers which, if developed, might achieve results which we now expect only from exceptional human beings. Therefore; be yourself. Hold up your head, throw back your shoulders; remember that the earth and all that is thereon belongs to you. Anyway, it is well to be inspired by such a thought. It is the proper mental attitude. Life is a hard battle, and the rewards are to the strong and courageous. Be inspired by the dominating determination to get all there is in your life. Develop all your capacities and powers to their utmost limit, and then you can rest assured, that every thought that stirs your soul will be up building rather than destructive in nature.

CHAPTER XXI: The Laugh Cure

The physiological effects of the mechanical and mental processes involved in laughing are not generally understood and appreciated. The "laugh cure" is a reality, for it is a remedy of very great value. Many a man, placed in a trying situation, would have been saved from tragic consequences if he could have found some means of arousing the emotions expressed in a good hearty laugh.

Naturally there may be times in life when a laugh is utterly impossible, or may seem so. Nevertheless the inclination to stimulate the emotions associated with laughter and good humor should be encouraged at every opportunity. There is no question that laughter has valuable vitalizing qualities. It undoubtedly adds to one's stamina. It gives one a hopeful spirit. It leads one to look upon the bright side of life. When you can laugh, the sun is shining regardless of how many clouds obscure the sky. No matter what other efforts you may be making to build strength and vitality, do not allow the serious aide of life to occupy you continuously.

Each day should have its laughing time, or its many laughing times. It is barely possible, of course, that laughing, like any other emotional expression, would become tiresome if overdone, but I am inclined to doubt the possibility of harmful effect under any circumstances. "All work and no play makes Jack a dull boy," and the relaxation and recuperation that go with laughing should be sought with a certain amount of regularity. If you cannot find recreation of this kind through any other source, then attend a "funny show." Go to a theater where merriment is supreme. On such occasions at least I would avoid tragedies or dramas that are inclined too much toward the sorrowful side of life. Personally, I have never had much use for plays of this sort. There are slough serious experiences in life without searching for recreation in the sorrows of others, which are, after all, only the expression of the imagination of some brooding dramatist. Some abnormal characters find pleasure in misery. I have heard some women say that "they enjoyed a good cry so much," and that "crying dramas were just grand." But I have been unable to discover anything

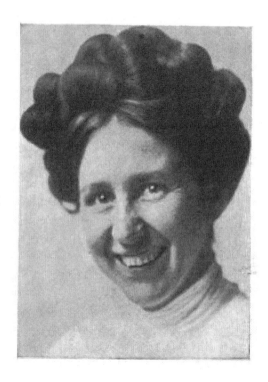

A smile that is worth while. Try this smile as a means of dispelling the "blues." You are sure to admit the superiority of the suggestion.

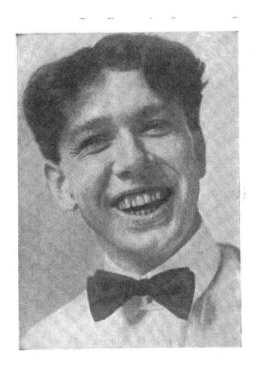

"The smile that won't come off." It is worth practicing to get this sort of smile. Try it in your mirror.

rational in such sentiments.

I may say, however, that in a sense there is a certain basis for this sentiment under certain circumstances. For crying, like laughter, has the physiological effect of producing a relaxation of tense nerves. There is a fundamental basis for crying, but this applies only to exceptional instances in which there is too much nervous tension. When nerves are strained to the "breaking point," crying will bring about a state of relaxation, and one will feel better. If there are times of strain when laughter is utterly impossible, then crying might even be beneficial. The effect on the breathing is very much the same in both cases, and there is a curious similarity in the action of the diaphragm and the mechanical character of the expulsion of the breath. Looking tat a person from behind, one cannot tell whether he is laughing or crying. Both produce relaxation of the nerves, both increase the activity of the lungs, and both involve a form of gymnastics for the diaphragm and entire breathing apparatus.

But, while crying offers relief from extreme tension or grief, it does not justify crying for the so-called pleasure derived from it. Laughter is a pleasure, in itself, as well as a symptom of merriment. It is the expression of keen, bounding joy. It is an emotive manifestation that stirs one's whole nature and vitalizes every part of the body. There is a sound, physiological basis for amusements that make us laugh. Taking the world over, incalculable sums of money are spent for amusements that make us laugh, and it is money well spent. It is a sound and healthy instinct that leads the tired business man or the tired laborer to seek for mirth-provoking recreations. Professional "funny men" like John Bunny and Charles Chaplin undoubtedly add to the health of the human race, and they add to the vitality of those in whom they stimulate laughter. I feel sorry for anyone who has lost the power to laugh freely and heartily. When a man has brooded so much over the sorrows and miseries of life that he can no longer laugh, his condition is indeed serious.

"Laugh and the world laughs with you; weep and you weep alone," is one of the truest things that Ella Wheeler Wilcox ever said. For a laugh

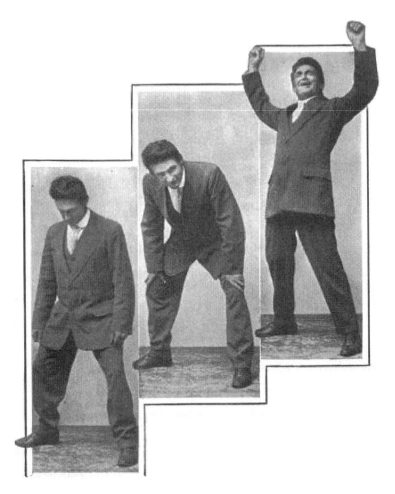

A mechanical means of producing laughter. Position in illustration at the left shows the beginning of this process. Stand with the feet wide apart and then bring the hands down with a vigorous slap just above the knees as shown in the central photograph. Now bring the bent arms upward and outward at the sides, as shown in the upper right-hand illustration, and proceed to make a noise as nearly like a laugh as possible. A repetition of this movement will soon get you in a "laughing humor." It is guaranteed to produce this result if you have an audience of one or more.

that is spontaneous and heartfelt is truly contagious, and in your little world, the circle of your friends, laughing brings a rich reward in increasing your own happiness as well as theirs.

The bodily expression and mechanical efforts that go with happiness will often induce the feelings and emotions associated therewith. To prove the accuracy of this statement, some morning when you are feeling especially gloomy and unpleasant, look into your mirror and go through the process of trying to make yourself smile. Screw up your features in such a manner as to force the required contractions of the facial muscles. If you continue your efforts long enough you will surely be rewarded by a real smile, and with the sense of good cheer that a smile will bring. You will make the surprising discovery at it is no longer an effort, for you will smile spontaneously.

To go even further try the laugh cure in the following manner. First of all assume a laughing position, in order to laugh properly and to secure the best results. Stand with feet far apart, and with the knees slightly bent. Now bring the palms of both hands down and "slap" them vigorously on the legs just above the knees, and then swing your bent arms overhead, making a noise as nearly as possible like laughing. Yes, you are quite right, it will sound very much like a cold stage laugh at first, and you will have to force it, but as you go on with the experiment it will gradually become more natural. Continue this long enough and I defy anyone to differentiate the emotions aroused from those associated with a real, spontaneous laugh.

In fact, if you have company while you are going through this process, I will guarantee that they will soon be "guffawing" loudly and violently. This experiment is an excellent one to thy on a company that is especially dull and in need of something unusual to awaken the spirit of good cheer.

CHAPTER XXII: Singing-The Great Tonic

Singing was designed by the Creator as a means of giving vent to joyous emotions. When one is overflowing with happiness it is entirely natural for him to break forth into song. Therefore when you sing the bodily mechanical efforts associated therewith are naturally inclined to arouse the mental attitude of joy, delight and allied emotions. I have already explained the tremendous value of certain bodily positions and mechanical efforts as a means of influencing the mental attitude. If singing is naturally the expression of joy, then by forcing oneself to sing when mentally downcast one encourages, and at times actually produces, happiness and good cheer.

But it is not only for its influence upon the mind that singing is valuable. It is a physical exercise requiring considerable effort. It wakes up the diaphragm. It promotes active circulation. It improves digestion. Therefore it has a double value for stimulating the physical as well as the mental functions. I would by all means encourage every inclination towards physical efforts of this sort.

Remember that the cultivation of the singing voice especially requires the expansion of the lungs. It means that breathing exercises of unusual value will be practiced diligently and persistently on every occasion that you exercise your vocal powers. It not only affects the lungs but the action of the diaphragm involved, and serves to massage, stimulate and invigorate the internal organs lying underneath. There is no need to dilate upon the value of exercise of this sort, for I have referred to this aspect of the question in a previous chapter.

If you have no special knowledge or training in the use of the singing voice, then simply do your best. Sing at every opportunity. If there is no music in your voice do not allow this to discourage you. Follow out the idea that singing is an exercise pure and simple. Let your friends understand that you are not impressed with your vocal ability, but that it is simply a form of exercise you take with religious regularity. Naturally if you can secure the opportunities associated with a musical education you are to be congratulated, and musical training largely devoted to vocal culture is far more valuable in its influence upon physical and mental powers than when limited to instrumental work.

Even apart from singing a good voice represents capital of great value. Any efforts that you make with a view to developing the singing voice will improve the speaking voice to a similar degree. Effective speakers do not always have musical voices, but all good singers possess good speaking voices. Therefore the work that you may do with a view to improving your singing voice will surely add to your vocal capital.

Furthermore, all the time spent in the development of your voice should be looked upon as a recreation. If you can make voice culture a hobby, so much the better. There is really no better means of taking one "away from oneself." You will find no more effective means of diversion from exhausting mental responsibilities, since you cannot think of something else while devoting your entire attention to singing.

Your mental attitude makes considerable difference in the results. Singing, as I have previously explained, is an expression of joy. To sing properly you should really be influenced by joyous emotions, and, though your musical efforts may be forced and mechanical in the beginning, you will usually find that the delight ordinarily associated with vocal expression will soon appear as a result of the physical and mechanical efforts involved in the training of the voice.

Naturally it is advisable to use the singing voice in the most advantageous manner, if possible, and it would therefore be well to secure the advice of competent instructors if you can, or at least to gain what helpful information there is in books on the subject. It is, of course, impossible to give any detailed advice in this short chapter, but I may say that I am engaged in the preparation of a book on vocal culture which will deal with the subject in an unusually practical manner. Voice culture, in many instances, is a mysterious and intricate study that even many of its teachers do not seem to understand in every detail. It is a notorious fact that many so-called vocal instructors, including some of the highest-priced members of the profession, frequently ruin magnificent voices by wrong methods of instruction. It is a simple matter to build up a good voice, but it is also a simple matter to ruin one by unnatural methods of training.

It is therefore well to learn to use the voice in a strictly natural manner, and without any straining or forcing of the tone. For instance, it is advisable to avoid any constriction of the muscles of the throat; that is to say, there should be no tension in the throat when singing. One should learn how to "place" the voice. Resonance is all-important.

Many really good teachers differ as to the proper methods of using the voice. Although there may be a reasonable excuse for a difference on some of the minor details of voice culture, yet there are certain fundamental principles upon which there should be a definite agreement, and it is these basic principles which will be presented in the book to which I have just referred.

At all events, whether or not you desire to take up vocal culture in a serious way, at least you should make it a point to sing at every opportunity. Break forth into song whenever the slightest excuse appears. If your voice is harsh, unpleasant and reminds your friends of a carpenter filing a saw, do not be discouraged. Every vocal artist had to make a beginning. No matter how bad your efforts may be you can probably recall voices that are still worse. Remember also that all voices improve with training. It is a matter of common agreement among instructors that anyone who possesses a speaking voice can also learn to sing. Anyway, at the worst, your hours of practice can be so arranged as to avoid annoying other people, or you can adopt a method that I have often used. For instance, when you are on a train, or in a busy center of the city in which there is a combination of noises which will drown your own voice, you can then sing or hum to your heart's content without annoying others. Remember that humming, if you carry it out with sufficient breath to produce real resonance, is practically as good as singing for the training of the voice.

There is one particular point of special value, and that is the advantage of singing when the stomach is empty. Vocal artists commonly refuse to sing immediately after eating. Your voice is free and full and clear when the stomach is empty. A few minutes of singing before each meal would enable one to digest his food far more satisfactorily. It would also establish the mental attitude best suited to perfect digestion.

Whenever you find responsibilities crowding upon you beyond your power to bear them, or when you realize that your mental attitude is sour, crabbed and pessimistic, then is the time to break forth into song. Nothing will bring about a pleasing change more quickly. Hum a tune. Sing some popular song. Put your soul into your efforts as much as possible, and you will literally be amazed at the value of this suggestion.

CHAPTER XXIII: The Daily Regimen

Following is a brief summary of the suggestions in this volume which may be incorporated in the daily regimen:

Rise from six to eight o'clock. Drink a cup of hot or cold water immediately upon arising.

Take the thyroid-stimulating exercises. Follow by spine-strengthening movements in combination with the hot-water-drinking.

Following these exercises a dry friction bath may be taken, if desired; also a cold bath. The latter is not necessary to the same extent while following the hot-water-drinking regimen as under ordinary circumstances. The bath may be varied from time to time by taking a cold sitz bath instead of a complete bath.

Before breakfast indulge in a good laugh or a little singing.

Eat a light breakfast-preferably consisting chiefly of acid fruits, such as oranges, apples, pears, grapefruit, grapes, etc.

Throughout the day while following your daily duties remember the suggestions in reference to proper position. Make a continuous and never-ending fight to keep a straight spine. Hold the chin in, down and backward, with spine erect as nearly as possible, whether sitting or standing.

Be hopeful, be cheerful, but cultivate the fighting spirit. You cannot have too much will power, determination.

Eat your first hearty meal between twelve and two o'clock, depending upon the time at which you had breakfast. From five to six hours should elapse between meals to insure perfect digestion. Masticate thoroughly. Enjoy your food as much as possible. Do not eat without a keen appetite.

Try to take a walk some time during the day. Remember during this walk to practice the thyroid-stimulating exercise-chin inward, downward and backward while holding a deep full breath, with the abdomen expanded.

Do not forget the necessity of using liquids freely. Have water close at hand so that your thirst can easily be satisfied.

Some time during the day, if possible, take some form of outdoor exercise which will compel deep full breathing similar to that induced by running.

Try to get a good laugh or do a little singing before your evening meal.

Your evening meal should be taken between six and eight o'clock, depending upon the time of breakfast and lunch. Do not forget my suggestion for closing the meal with a little acid fruit. A few spinal exercises, a walk or a short run before retiring can be highly recommended.

During the evening, if convenient, take an air bath.

Take a combination sun bath and air bath in the morning or at any time during the day that is convenient. If you cannot take a regular sun bath wear light-colored clothing and walk on the sunny side of the street when outdoors to get the sun's rays through your clothing.

Take a hot soap-and-water bath once or twice a week.

Retire early enough to awake thoroughly refreshed at proper rising time without the warning of an alarm clock.

For more old time classics of strength, visit:

STRONGMANBOOKS.COM

Sign up on the website for a free gift and
for updates about new books added regularly.

Title Available from Authors including:

Arthur Saxon

Maxick

George F. Jowett

Otto Arco

Eugene Sandow

Bob Hoffman and the York Company

George Hackenschmidt

Edward Aston

Bernarr MacFadden

Earle Liederman

Alan Calvert

Alexander Zass

Monte Saldo

and more...

Made in the USA
Las Vegas, NV
08 January 2024

84075938R00113